AF879887

Acta Hæmatologica

Founded 1948 by E. Meulengracht, K. Rohr, and G. Rosenow
Continued by H. Lüdin (1960–1977), U. Bucher (1977–1983), R.S. Hillman (1978–1987), H.R. Marti (1983–1988), E.A. Beck (1984–1988), B. Ramot (1989–1995)

KARGER

Printed in Switzerland
on acid-free paper by
Reinhardt Druck, Basel

Appears 6-weekly:
2 volumes per year
(8 issues)

Guidelines for Authors

Acta Hæmatologica

Submission

Manuscripts written in English should be submitted using the online submission website at:

www.karger.com/aha

or as an e-mail attachment (the preferred word-processing package is MS-Word) to the Editorial Office:

aha@karger.ch

Prof. I. Ben-Bassat
S. KARGER AG
Editorial Office Acta Haematologica
PO Box
CH–4009 Basel (Switzerland)

All manuscripts must be accompanied by a covering letter signed by all authors. Assurance should be given that the manuscript is not under simultaneous consideration by any other publication. The preferred word processing package is Word for Windows®. Presentation of manuscripts should conform with the Uniform Requirements for Manuscripts Submitted to Biomedical Journals (see N Engl J Med 1997;336:309–315).

Conditions

All manuscripts are subject to editorial review. Manuscripts are received with the explicit understanding that they are not under simultaneous consideration by any other publication. Submission of an article for publication implies the transfer of the copyright from the author to the publisher upon acceptance. Accepted papers become the permanent property of 'Acta Haematologica' and may not be reproduced by any means, in whole or in part, without the written consent of the publisher. It is the author's responsibility to obtain permission to reproduce illustrations, tables, etc. from other publications.

Arrangement

Recommendation for Usage of Units and Abbreviations: The Editorial Board of 'Acta Haematologica' supports the recommendations of the 'International Committee for Standardization in Hematology' for using the SI (Système International d'Unités) equivalents in haematological literature. The standard abbreviations used for measurements of weight, length, volume, and time (i.e. mg, cm, ml, min) are used without definition. The abbreviations listed on the opposite page also require no definition. Please note that punctuation is not needed. When using other abbreviations, spell out the name in full at the first mention, and follow with the abbreviation in parentheses.

Title page: The first page of each paper should indicate the title, the authors' names, the institute where the work was conducted, and a short title for use as running head.

Full address: The exact postal address of the corresponding author complete with postal code must be given at the bottom of the title page. Please also supply phone and fax numbers, as well as e-mail address.

Key words: For indexing purposes, a list of 3–10 key words in English is essential.

Abstract: Each paper needs an abstract of up to 10 lines.

Footnotes: Avoid footnotes. When essential, they are numbered consecutively and typed at the foot of the appropriate page.

Tables and illustrations: Tables and illustrations (both numbered in Arabic numerals) should be prepared on separate sheets. Tables require a heading and figures a legend, also prepared on a separate sheet. For the reproduction of illustrations, only good drawings and original photographs can be accepted; negatives or photocopies cannot be used. Due to technical reasons, figures with a screen background should not be submitted. When possible, group several illustrations on one block for reproduction (max. size 180 × 223 mm) or provide crop marks. On the back of each illustration, indicate its number, the author's name, and 'top' with a soft pencil. Electronically submitted b/w halftone and color illustrations must have a final resolution of 300 dpi after scaling, line drawings one of 800–1,200 dpi.

Color illustrations: Up to 6 color illustrations per page can be integrated within the text at the special price of CHF/USD 660.00 per page. Color illustrations are reproduced at the author's expense.

References: In the text identify references by Arabic numerals [in square brackets]. Material submitted for publication but not yet accepted should be noted as 'unpublished data' and not be included in the reference list. The list of references should include only those publications which are cited in the text. Do not alphabetize; number references in the order in which they are first mentioned in the text. The surnames of the authors followed by initials should be given. There should be no punctuation other than a comma to separate the authors. Please cite all authors, 'et al' is not sufficient. Abbreviate journal names according to the Index Medicus system. (Also see International Committee of Medical Journal Editors: Uniform requirements for manuscripts submitted to biomedical journals. N Engl J Med 1997;336:309–315.)

Digital Object Identifier (DOI)
S. Karger Publishers supports DOIs as unique identifiers for articles. A DOI number will be printed on the title page of each article. DOIs can be useful in the future for identifying and citing articles published online without volume or issue information. More information can be found at www.doi.org.

Examples
(a) Papers published in periodicals: Sun J, Koto H, Chung KF: Interaction of ozone and allergen challenges on bronchial responsiveness and inflammation in sensitised guinea pigs. Int Arch Allergy Immunol 1997;112:191–195.
(b) Papers published only with DOI numbers: Theoharides TC, Boucher W, Spear K: Serum interleukin-6 reflects disease severity and osteoporosis in mastocytosis patients. Int Arch Allergy Immunol DOI: 10.1159/000063858.
(c) Monographs: Matthews DE, Farewell VT: Using and Understanding Medical Statistics, ed 3, revised. Basel, Karger, 1996.
(d) Edited books: Parren PWHI, Burton DR: Antibodies against HIV-1 from phage display libraries: Mapping of an immune response and progress towards antiviral immunotherapy; in Capra JD (ed): Antibody Engineering. Chem Immunol. Basel, Karger, 1997, vol 65, pp 18–56.

Page Charges

Authors are charged CHF/USD 145.00 per printed page for the first 6 pages and CHF/USD 290.00 for each additional page, including tables, illustrations, and references. 1 printed page is equal to approximately 3 manuscript pages.

Rapid Communication

Manuscripts intended for rapid communication must present new findings of sufficient importance to justify their accelerated acceptance. They should follow the general arrangement of research papers except that the separate sections should not be formally titled. They should not be more than three pages in length (including figures, tables and references). Proofs are checked by the Main Editor and not sent to the authors. Review will be rapid, and once accepted, the paper will be included in the next planned issue. If manuscripts require significant change after editing they will be treated as brief communications and returned to the authors for correction.

Brief Communication

The general arrangement for brief communications is the same as for research papers except that the manuscript is not divided into separate sections formally entitled introduction, methods, results, discussion. No abstract is required. These should not be more than 3 pages in length.

Letter to the Editor

Comments and responses to previously published articles and other short correspondences are welcome. They should be limited to 1 or $1^1/_2$ manuscript pages with a general arrangement as specified for Brief Communications.

Galley Proofs

Unless indicated otherwise, galley proofs are sent to the first-named author and should be returned with the least possible delay. Alterations made in galley proofs, other than the correction of printer's errors, are charged to the author. No page proofs are supplied.

Reprints

Order forms and a price list are sent with the galley proofs. Orders submitted after the issue is printed are subject to considerably higher prices.

KARGER

Fax +41 61 306 12 34
E-Mail karger@karger.ch
www.karger.com

The Guidelines for Authors are available at:
www.karger.com/aha_Guidelines

General Information

Acta Haematologica

Publication data: 'Acta Haematologica' is published 8 times a year. Volumes 115–116, each with 4 issues, appear in 2006.

Subscription rates: Subscriptions run for a full calendar year. Prices are given per year.
Personal subscription:

Print or Online	Print/Online combined
CHF 879.–	CHF 969.–
EUR 651.–	EUR 717.–
USD 799.00	USD 881.00
postage and handling	(added to print and print/online)
CHF 44.80 Europe,	CHF 66.40 Overseas
EUR 32.40	
USD 60.80	

Institutional subscription:

Print or Online	Print/Online combined
CHF 1758.–	CHF 1898.–
EUR 1302.–	EUR 1406.–
USD 1598.00	USD 1726.00
postage and handling	(added to print and print/online)
CHF 56.00 Europe,	CHF 83.20 Overseas
EUR 40.40	
USD 76.00	

Airmail surcharge: CHF 56.00 / USD 50.80
Discount subscription prices:
International Society of Haematology

Microforms: Please direct all enquiries and orders to:
University Microfilms Inc.
300 North Zeeb Road, P.O. Box 1346
Ann Arbor, MI 48106-1346 (USA)

Subscription orders: Orders can be placed at agencies, bookstores, directly with the Publisher
S. Karger AG, P.O. Box
CH–4009 Basel (Switzerland)
or with any of the following distributors:
Deutschland: S. Karger GmbH, Postfach
D–79095 Freiburg
France: Librairie Luginbühl
36, bd de Latour-Maubourg
F–75007 Paris
Great Britain, Ireland: S. Karger AG
4 Rickett Street
London SW6 1RU, UK
USA: S. Karger Publishers, Inc.
26 West Avon Road, P.O. Box 529
Farmington, CT 06085, USA
India, Bangladesh, Sri Lanka:
Panther Publishers Private Ltd.
33, First Main
Koramangala First Block
Bangalore 560 034, India
Japan: Karger Japan, Inc.
Yushima S Bld. 3F
4-2-3, Yushima, Bunkyo-ku
Tokyo 113-0034, Japan

Change of address: Both old and new address should be sent to the subscription source.

Single issues and back volumes: Information can be obtained through the Publisher.

Advertising: Correspondence and rate requests should be addressed to the Publisher.

Bibliographic indices: This journal is regularly listed in bibliographic services, including *Current Contents®* and Index Medicus/MEDLINE.

Book Reviews: Books are accepted for review by special agreement.

Usage of Units and Abbreviations

Entity	Abbreviation	Recommended SI equivalent	Not recommended
Red blood cell count	RBC	$10^{12}/l$	$10^6/mm^3$
White blood cell count	WBC	$10^9/l$	$10^3/mm^3$
Platelet count		... × $10^9/l$	... × $10^3/mm^3$
Reticulocyte count		% (or ... × $10^9/l$)	% (or ../mm^3)
Haemoglobin	Hb	g/dl[a]	g/100 ml
Packed cell volume	PCV	ratio[b]	%
Mean cell volume	MCV	fl	
Mean cell haemoglobin	MCH	pg	
Mean cell haemoglobin concentration	MCHC	g/dl	%
Mean cell diameter	MCD	μm	
Sedimentation rate	ESR	mm in 1 h[c]	
Plasma haemoglobin	Plasma Hb	mg/l	μg/100 ml
Serum vitamin B12		ng/l	
Serum folate		μg/l	
Serum iron		μmol/l	μg/100 ml
Total iron binding capacity	TIBC	μmol/l	μg/100 ml
Unsaturated iron binding capacity	UIBC	μmol/l	μg/100 ml
Transferrin		g/l	mg/100 ml
Serum haptoglobin		g/l	mg/100 ml
Plasma fibrinogen		g/l	mg/100 ml

a The concentration for Hb only is expressed as ../dl and not ../l or ../100 ml.
b No unit necessary, 1/1 is implied.
c Indicate method only if other than Westergren.

KARGER

Fax +41 61 306 12 34
E-Mail karger@karger.ch
www.karger.com

The Journal Home Page is available at:
www.karger.com/aha

F 06350

Acta Hæmatologica

Issues of Haemostasis and Thrombosis in Children

Guest Editors
Gili Kenet, Tel Hashomer
Ulrike Nowak-Göttl, Münster

26 figures, 2 in color, and 30 tables, 2006

KARGER

Basel · Freiburg · Paris · London · New York ·
Bangalore · Bangkok · Singapore · Tokyo · Sydney

S. Karger
Medical and Scientific Publishers
Basel • Freiburg • Paris • London
New York • Bangalore • Bangkok
Singapore • Tokyo • Sydney

Disclaimer
The statements, options and data contained in this publication are solely those of the individual authors and contributors and not of the publisher and the editor(s). The appearance of advertisements in the journal is not a warranty, endorsement, or approval of the products or services advertised or of their effectiveness, quality or safety. The publisher and the editor(s) disclaim responsibility for any injury to persons or property resulting from any ideas, methods, instructions or products referred to in the content or advertisements.

Drug Dosage
The authors and the publisher have exerted every effort to ensure that drug selection and dosage set forth in this text are in accord with current recommendations and practice at the time of publication. However, in view of ongoing research, changes in government regulations, and the constant flow of information relating to drug therapy and drug reactions, the reader is urged to check the package insert for each drug for any change in indications and dosage and for added warnings and precautions. This is particularly important when the recommended agent is a new and/or infrequently employed drug.

Printed in Switzerland on acid-free paper by
Reinhardt Druck, Basel
ISBN 3–8055–8098–3

KARGER

Fax +41 61 306 12 34
E-Mail karger@karger.ch
www.karger.com

Vol. 115, No. 3–4, 2006

Acta Hæmatologica

Contents

KARGER

Fax +41 61 306 12 34
E-Mail karger@karger.ch
www.karger.com

Access to full text and tables of contents, including tentative ones for forthcoming issues: www.karger.com/aha_issues

Editorial

Acta Haematologica

Acta Haematol 2006;115:137–140
DOI: 10.1159/000090926

Bleeding and Thrombosis Issues in Pediatric Patients: Current Approach to Diagnosis and Treatment

Gili Kenet[a] Ulrike Nowak-Göttl[b]

[a]Pediatric Coagulation Service, National Hemophilia Center and Institute of Thrombosis and Hemostasis, Sheba Medical Center, Tel Hashomer, Israel; [b]Department of Paediatric Haematology and Oncology, University of Münster, Münster, Germany

Hemostasis is a dynamic process which begins in utero. Coagulation factors are synthesized by fetuses by 10 weeks' gestational age and their concentrations gradually increase, being physiologically lower in premature infants as compared to full-term babies or healthy children [1–4].

In the neonate, plasma concentrations of vitamin K-dependent coagulation factors (II, VII, IX, X) and contact factors (XI, XII, prekallikrein and high-molecular-weight kininogen) are about 50% of adult values [4]. Furthermore, the capacity of newborns to generate thrombin, dependent upon plasma concentrations of procoagulants, is reduced [5, 6]. These facts, theoretically increasing the risk of severe bleeding, are balanced by the protective effects of physiological deficiencies of the inhibitors of coagulation, as well as by the decreased fibrinolytic capacity in infants [4, 7].

In this special issue Chan and his colleagues discuss the phenomenon of reduced plasmin generation in neonates as compared to adults and the lower inhibitory antifibrinolytic effect of lipoprotein on neonatal as compared to adult plasma. The latter may stem from physiologically reduced plasminogen concentrations. Decreased neonatal fibrinolysis potentially increases the risk of perinatal thrombosis, which may require the use of thrombolytic therapy.

The clinical presentation of bleeding disorders in infants is characterized by one or more of the following symptoms: cephalhematomas, injury-related bleeding and bleeding into the skin, manifesting as petechiae, purpura and ecchymoses. Persistent oozing from the umbilical stump is typical for infants with defective fibrinogen production or function and FXIII deficiency. Joint hemarthroses, typical for severe hemophilias, rarely occur before ambulation. A small proportion of infants with severe coagulation factor deficiencies may present with intracranial hemorrhage as the first manifestation [8–10].

Laboratory variations of hemostatic tests may make it difficult to establish any diagnosis of bleeding disorder in infants [1–4].

Diagnostic problems of special concern are the need to adapt all coagulation assays for small amounts of blood and the age-related interpretation required for test results. The prolonged PT in neonates reflects decreased plasma concentrations of vitamin K-dependent factors, whereas the prolonged PTT stems from decreased plasma levels of contact factors as well [2–4]. The levels of FVIII, FV and FXIII correlate well with adult boundaries. Plasma concentrations of fibrinogen may be skewed upwards, despite the fact that thrombin clotting time may be prolonged, due to a normally present 'fetal' fibrinogen [11]. Bleeding time is shorter in healthy neonates as compared to adults, probably because of increased concentrations and enhanced function of von Willebrand factor (VWF) and VWF large multimers [2–4, 12], increased hematocrit and the presence of large red cells. The platelet num-

KARGER

Fax +41 61 306 12 34
E-Mail karger@karger.ch
www.karger.com

0001–5792/06/1154–0137$23.50/0

Accessible online at:
www.karger.com/aha

Gili Kenet, MD
Pediatric Coagulation Service, National Hemophilia Center and
Institute of Thrombosis and Hemostasis, Sheba Medical Center
Tel Hashomer, 52621 (Israel)
Tel. +972 3 530 2120, Fax +972 3 535 1806, E-Mail gili.kenet@sheba.health.gov.il

ber of neonates is within adult limits; however, the evaluation of platelet function is difficult and deserves special attention. Neonatal platelets were found to be hyporeactive in some studies. Some of the reasons reported are decreased receptors, deficient thromboxane synthesis and impaired signal transduction [8, 13, 14]. In this special issue Yael Levy-Shraga and her colleagues report the use of a modified, relatively new technique and device, the cone and platelet analyzer (CPA) as a rapid, feasible mode to assess shear-induced neonatal platelet aggregation. CPA values of preterm and term infants tested in whole cord blood correlated with gestational age; however, the clinical correlation and the predictive value of the test remain to be elucidated. Maayan-Metzger et al. in their manuscript aimed at defining the impact of maternal selective serotonin reuptake inhibitor therapy that may potentially impair platelet function of neonates, using CPA platelet function tests to compare the neonates of treated mothers versus controls; neither bleeding manifestations nor platelet function CPA impairments were found in this study.

Among severe congenital factor deficiencies the representative and mostly reported disorder is hemophilia. Children with hemophilia may present with variable bleeding tendencies requiring a 'tailored' therapeutic approach [15, 16]. In the review by Amy Dunn and Thomas Abshire therapy considerations in children with hemophilia are discussed, including a description of coagulation factor concentrates currently available and suggestive guidelines for prophylactic therapy. Guy Young, in another manuscript of our special issue, reflects on the challenge of treating hemophilia patients with inhibitors. Inhibitor prevention is discussed and therapy with bypassing agents and novel drugs for bleeding episodes as well as prophylaxis is suggested with potential modes of monitoring treatment outcome.

Prenatal diagnosis of most severe congenital factor deficiencies is currently possible. Thus in families with a history of hemophilia prevention is available since fetal DNA, obtained through amniocentesis or chorionic villi biopsy, can be tested for the presence of known mutations or analyzed to compare linkage and sequences against the sick patient and his parents. Early diagnosis allows for termination of pregnancy or proceeding towards early intervention and therapy, as indicated. With regard to future perspectives, the progress of gene therapy trials may yield the best answer for hemophilia within a few years.

Venous and arterial thrombosis are increasingly diagnosed and reported in children. Due to the special properties of the pediatric hemostatic system, thrombotic manifestation occurs in 0.07/10,000 children, 5.3/10,000 pediatric hospital admissions, and 2.4/1,000 admissions of newborns to intensive care units. Neonates are at the highest risk of thromboembolic complications as compared to older children, with a reported annual incidence of 0.5/10,000 live births in Caucasian children, possibly due to the lower concentrations of the physiological inhibitors of the coagulation system along with their markedly reduced fibrinolytic capacity [17, 18]. The incidence of vascular accidents decreases significantly after the first year of life, with a second peak during puberty and adolescence again associated with reduced fibrinolytic activity [17].

Numerous clinical and environmental conditions, such as peripartal asphyxia, neonatal infections, fetal diabetes, the use of central lines, trauma or surgery, dehydration, malignant diseases, renal diseases, autoimmune diseases, obesity, immobilization, or the intake of oral contraceptives by adolescent girls may result in elevated thrombin generation with subsequent thrombus formation. In addition, various genetic prothrombotic defects, particularly those affecting the physiological anticoagulant systems (antithrombin, protein C and protein S deficiencies, the mutation G1691A of coagulation factor V, and the factor II G20210A gene variant) have been established as risk factors for thrombotic events in the white pediatric population [19–24]. Furthermore, moderate hyperhomocysteinemia as well as increased concentrations of lipoprotein (a) and factor VIII have recently been shown to significantly enhance the risk of thromboembolic arterial and venous thrombosis in pediatric and adult patients [25–27]. Nevertheless, until today up to 30–40% of pediatric patients with symptomatic thromboembolism do not have any identifiable inherited prothrombotic risk factor. Therefore, studies dealing with the association between hemostatic factors and pediatric thromboembolism are of special interest. In this special pediatric issue, population-based data on arterial ischemic stroke and cerebral venous thrombosis in children were summarized by Mariana Bonduell et al. based on a 12-year Argentinean pediatric thrombosis registry. The authors report on underlying inherited and acquired conditions, mortality and recurrence data, as well as clinical outcome rates. Burghaus and co-authors describe in a case-control study that elevated α_1-antitrypsin increases the risk of arterial ischemic stroke in white children 4.0-fold independently from other established thrombophilias. In this controlled study cutoff values above the age-dependent 90th percentiles were derived from 229 healthy controls. Danckwardt and co-workers review the pathomechanism of clinically relevant mutations in the factor II gene, which may promote further understanding of the etiology of pediatric thromboembolism.

In a further manuscript dealing with thrombosis epidemiology in selective pediatric high-risk groups, Cyr and colleagues studied the incidence of deep vein thrombosis in children after major trauma. The authors report an incidence of 3.3 per 1,000 admissions diagnosed with symptomatic deep vein thrombosis. In this Canadian cohort thrombosis was more common in older children with high injury severity scores, in patients with thoracic injuries, in children suffering spinal injuries, and in subjects with central venous lines. Shoshana Revel-Vilk reviews central venous line thromboses, comprising a significant risk of venous thromboembolism in pediatric patients. Interestingly, catheter thrombosis in children may be missed, since its reported frequency is as low as 5% in studies including only symptomatic cases and as high as 50% in studies where patients are systematically screened for catheter-related thrombosis. The review describes risk factors for catheter-related thrombosis that may be associated with the methods used for catheter insertion as well as individual patient characteristics, and reflects upon diagnosis and treatment.

Postthrombotic syndrome is a definition used to determine thrombotic sequelae in adult patients with deep vein thrombosis. However, it also is increasingly noted in pediatric patients. In her review, Marilyn Manco-Johnson focuses on postthrombotic syndrome in children, highlighting functional tools which can be used in order to accurately assess this problem. In addition, Leo Brandão and his group from Canada report on the specific findings of postthrombotic syndrome following upper limb system thrombosis, mainly occurring in adolescents.

The management of children with acute thrombosis usually comprises therapy with anticoagulants [28, 29]. Thrombolytic agents may be used during acute thrombotic events, and are currently mainly applied in neonates [30], due to the physiologically reduced fibrinolytic capacity of this age group [18]. In pediatric patients with thrombosis, however, antithrombotic treatment protocols cannot automatically be adjusted from adults. In this issue Nick Merkel and colleagues report on a long-term pilot study in pediatric patients with venous thrombosis treated with enoxaparin. In this survey enoxaparin was prescribed twice daily in children, and was found to be safe and effective, especially when the drug was administered over a mean period of time of 10 months. One of the major adverse effects of heparin treatment, heparin-induced thrombocytopenia, is well known and may complicate antithrombotic therapy. This severe adverse effect of heparin is more common in adults and has rarely been reported in children. Bidlingmaier and colleagues review the literature available for heparin-induced thrombocytopenia in pediatric patients, including treatment regiments applied in this cohort so far.

Long-term anticoagulant therapy may be required for selected pediatric patients in order to prevent a recurrence of thrombosis [31]. The potentially protective role of secondary prophylaxis in high-risk conditions also deserves further attention in the future.

In summary, the current manuscripts collected in our special issue on pediatric coagulation highlight some of the controversies associated with diagnosis, epidemiology and therapy of bleeding disorders as well as thrombosis in children. Prospective randomized multicenter trials and data collection are warranted in order to improve the understanding and treatment of these disorders.

References

1 Reverdiau-Moalic P, Delahousse B, Body G, Bardos GBP, Delahousse B, Leroy J, Gruel Y: Evolution of blood coagulation activators and inhibitors in the healthy human fetus. Blood 1996;88:900–906.

2 Andrew M, Paes B, Milner R, Johnston M, Mitchell L, Tollefsen DM, Castle V, Powers P: Development of the human coagulation system in the healthy premature infant. Blood 1988;72:1651–1657.

3 Andrew M, Paes B, Johnston M: Development of the hemostatic system in the neonate and young infant. Am J Pediatr Hematol Oncol 1990;12:95–104.

4 Andrew M, Vegh P, Johnston M, Bowker J, Ofosu F, Mitchell L: Maturation of the hemostatic system during childhood. Blood 1992; 80:1998–2005.

5 Cvirm G, Gallistl S, Muntean W: Effects of antithrombin and protein C on thrombin generation in newborn and adult plasma. Thromb Res 1999;93:183–190.

6 Andrew M, Schmidt B, Mitchell L, Paes B, Ofosu F: Thrombin generation in newborn plasma is critically dependent on the concentration of prothrombin. Thromb Haemost 1990;63:27–30.

7 Summaria L: Comparison of human normal, full-term, fetal and adult plasminogen by physical and chemical analyses. Haemostasis 1989; 19:266–273.

8 Yoffe G, Buchanan GR: Intracranial hemorrhage in newborn and young infants with hemophilia. J Pediatr 1988;113:333.

9 Abbondanzo SL, Gootenbeg JE, Lofts R, McPherson R: Intracranial hemorrhage in congenital deficiency of FXIII. Am J Pediatr Hematol Oncol 1988;10:65–68.

10 Struwe FE: Intracranial hemorrhage and occlusive hydrocephalus in hereditary bleeding disorders. Dev Med Child Neurol 1970;12: 165.

11 Witt I, Muller H, Kunter LJ: Evidence for the existence of fetal fibrinogen. Thromb Diath Haemorrh 1969;22:101–109.
12 Katz JA, Moake JL, McPherson PD, Weinstein MJ, Moise KJ, Carpenter RJ, Sala DJ: Relationship between human development and disappearance of unusually large von Willebrand factor multimers from plasma. Blood 1989;73:1851–1858.
13 Rajasekar D, Bernard M, Francis J Bednarek F: Platelet hyporeactivity in very low birth weight neonates. Thromb Haemost 1997;77: 1002–1007.
14 Israels SJ, Odaibo FS, Robertson C, McMillan EM, McNicol A: Deficient thromboxane synthesis and response in platelets from premature infants. Pediatr Res 1997;41:218–223.
15 Brettlet D, Levine P: Clinical manifestations and therapy of inherited coagulation factor deficiencies; in Colman RW, Hirsh J, Marder VJ, Salzman EW (eds): Hemostasis and Thrombosis: Basic Principles and Clinical Practice, ed 3. Philadelphia, Lippincott, 1999, pp 169–183.
16 Astermark J, Petrini P, Tengborn L, Schulman S, Ljung R, Berntorp E: Primary prophylaxis in severe haemophilia should be started at an early age but can be individualized. Br J Haematol 1999;105:1109–1113.
17 Andrew M: Developmental hemostasis: relevance to thromboembolic complications in pediatric patients. Thromb Haemost 1995;74: 415–425.
18 Reis M, Klinge J, Rauch R: Age-related reference values for activation markers of the coagulation and fibrinolytic systems in children. Thromb Res 1997;85:341–344.
19 Schmidt B, Andrew M: Neonatal thrombosis: report of a prospective Canadian and international registry. Pediatrics 1995;96:939–943.
20 van Ommen CH, Heijboer H, Buller HR, Hirasing RA, Heijmans HS, Peters M: Venous thromboembolism in childhood: a prospective 2-year registry in the Netherlands. J Pediatr 2001;139:676–681.
21 Heller C, Schobess R, Kurnik K, Junker R, Gunther G, Kreuz W, Nowak-Gottl U: Abdominal venous thrombosis in neonates and infants: role of prothrombotic risk factors – a multi-center case-control study. Br J Haematol 2000;111:534–539.
22 Revel-Vilk S, Chan A, Bauman M, Massicotte P: Prothrombotic conditions in an unselected cohort of children with venous thromboembolic disease. J Thromb Haemost 2003;1:915–921.
23 Ehrenforth S, Junker R, Koch HG, Kreuz W, Munchow N, Scharrer I, Nowak-Gottl U: Multicenter evaluation of combined prothrombotic defects with thrombophilia in childhood. Eur J Pediatr 1999;158:S97–S104.
24 Kenet G, Sadetzki S, Murad H, Martinowitz U, Rosenberg N, Gitel S, Rechavi G, Inbal A: Factor V Leiden and antiphospholipid antibodies are significant risk factors for ischemic stroke in children. Stroke 2000;31:1283–1288.
25 van Beynum IM, Smeitnik JA, den Heijer M, te Poele Pothoff MT, Blom HJ: Hyperhomocysteinemia: a risk for ischemic stroke in children. Circulation 1999;99:2070–2072.
26 Nowak-Gottl U, Junker P, Hartmeier M, Koch HG, Munchow N, Assmann G, von Eckardstein A: Increased lipoprotein (a) is an important risk factor for venous thrombosis in childhood. Circulation 1999;100:743–748.
27 Goldenberg NA, Knapp-Clevenger R, Manco-Johnson M: Elevated plasma factor VIII and D-dimer levels as predictors of poor outcome of thrombosis in children. N Engl J Med 2004; 351:1081–1088.
28 Andrew M, Michelson AD, Bovill E, Leaker M, Massicotte MP: Guidelines for antithrombotic therapy in pediatric patients. J Pediatr 1998; 132:575–588.
29 Dix D, Andrew M, Marzinotto V, Charpentier K, Bridge S, Monagle P, deVeber G, Leaker M, Chan AK, Massicotte MP: The use of low molecular weight heparin in pediatric patients: a prospective cohort study. J Pediatr 2000;136: 439–445.
30 Nowak-Gottl U, Auberger K, Halimeh S, Junker R, Klinge J, Kreuz WD, Ries M, Schlegel N: Thrombolysis in newborns and infants. Thromb Haemost 1999;82:S112–S116.
31 Kurnik K, Koch A, Strater R, Schobess R, Heller C, Nowak-Gottl U: Recurrent thromboembolism in infants and children suffering from symptomatic neonatal arterial stroke: a prospective follow-up study. Stroke 2003;34: 2887–2892.

Acta Haematologica

Acta Haematol 2006;115:141–151
DOI: 10.1159/000090927

The Influence of Age on in vitro Plasmin Generation in the Presence of Fibrin Monomer

Nagina Parmar[a] Lesley G. Mitchell[a] Leslie R. Berry[c,d] Maureen Andrew[b] Anthony K.C. Chan[b–d]

[a]Pediatric Thrombosis and Hemostasis Program and [b]Department of Hematology/Oncology, The Hospital for Sick Children, Toronto; [c]Henderson Research Centre and [d]Department of Pediatrics, McMaster University, Hamilton, Canada

Key Words

Endothelial cells · Fibrin · Plasmin · Plasminogen

Abstract

Background and Objectives: The components of the fibrinolytic system interact to generate plasmin from its zymogen form, plasminogen. At birth, all the components of the fibrinolytic system are present but with differing plasma concentrations. The present study was undertaken to explore the effect of physiological, age-dependent factors of the fibrinolytic system during childhood on the capacity to generate plasmin. ***Design and Methods:*** Total plasmin generation was measured in venous plasma from umbilical cords and adults, on plastic and cell surfaces, in the presence of fibrin monomer, Desafib. Plasminogen, its inhibitors α_2-antiplasmin and plasminogen activator inhibitor type 1, and plasmin-α_2-antiplasmin complex in the time samples were assayed by enzyme-linked immunosorbent assay. The effect of addition of plasminogen on the plasmin generation in cord plasma and the effect of lipoprotein on adult and cord plasmin generation were measured. ***Results:*** On the surface of human umbilical vein endothelial cells, onset of plasmin generation was earlier (40 min) compared to plastic (60 min) but total plasmin generation was similar on both surfaces. The addition of plasminogen to cord plasma increased plasmin generation. Supplementation of lipoprotein in adult plasma had an inhibitory effect, but there was no significant effect in cord plasma. ***Interpretations and Conclusions:*** Plasmin generation is reduced in newborn compared to adult plasma. Decreased plasmin generation in cord plasma is likely due to decreased plasminogen concentration. The antifibrinolytic effect of lipoprotein is more pronounced in adults as compared to newborns due to the presence of higher plasminogen concentration.

Introduction

The fibrinolytic system is closely linked to the coagulation system, and the balance between the two systems determines the formation and extent of thrombi in response to endothelial injury [1]. There are age-related, biologically important, differences in both the coagulation system and fibrinolytic system at birth and throughout childhood [2]. At birth, all components of the fibrinolytic system are present but with differing plasma concentrations of key components and evidence of significant, transient activation with plasmin generation [3]. In gen-

KARGER

Fax +41 61 306 12 34
E-Mail karger@karger.ch
www.karger.com

0001–5792/06/1154–0141$23.50/0

Accessible online at:
www.karger.com/aha

Anthony K.C. Chan
Henderson Research Center, 711 Concession Street
Hamilton, ON L8V 1C3 (Canada)
Tel. +1 905 527 2299, ext. 43559, Fax +1 905 575 2646
E-Mail achan@thrombosis.hhscr.org

eral, components of the fibrinolytic system include plasminogen, plasminogen activators [tissue plasminogen activator (tPA) and urokinase plasminogen activator (uPA)], inhibitors [plasminogen activator inhibitor type 1 (PAI-1), α_2-antiplasmin (α_2AP), α_2-macroglobulin (α_2M)] and thrombin activatable fibrinolysis inhibitor. Fibrin-bound tPA interacts with plasminogen to generate plasmin [4, 5], which in turn cleaves fibrin to form soluble degradation products [6]. Interactions with the coagulation cascade impact on this fibrinolytic system since plasminogen activation can be promoted by elevated levels of active tPA resulting from complexation of PAI-1 inhibitor with activated protein C [7–9]. Once formed, plasmin reacts with α_2AP to form a 1:1 stoichiometric complex that has no further enzymatic activity. Alternatively, plasmin can bind to α_2M and then cleave a bait region of this inhibitor, resulting in a conformational change which traps the proteinase without decreasing its activity against small molecules (such as chromogenic substrates) [4]. Thus, the large fibrin molecule cannot access the active site of plasmin complexed to α_2M [7].

More recently, it has been shown that plasmin generation is increased by the binding of plasminogen and tPA to fibrin [10–12] and to endothelial cell surfaces [13]. Fibrin affects protease-inhibitor interactions by two distinct mechanisms. Firstly, fibrin protects proteases from their inhibitors. Thus, fibrin-bound plasmin resists inactivation, whereas fluid phase activity is inhibited by α_2AP, resulting in a half-life for the fibrinolytic molecule of only about 0.1 s [14]. Secondly, fibrin promotes interaction between tPA and its substrate plasminogen, thereby enhancing tPA activity [10, 12]. In particular, free tPA has significant affinity for fibrin, mediated through lysine binding sites. Although the conversion of plasminogen to plasmin is accelerated by binding of plasminogen and tPA to fibrin, recent evidence suggests that the endothelium plays a significant role in the generation and regulation of plasmin [12]. Fibrin binds to an endothelial surface-localized system [15] while endothelial-produced tPA is expressed on the plasma membrane and secreted onto the extracellular matrix [16] or into the circulation [17, 18]. Overall, binding of fibrin [15, 19], plasminogen [13, 20] and tPA [20] or uPA [20, 21] to endothelial surfaces accelerates plasmin generation.

The age-dependent physiological differences of the fibrinolytic system in the young (reduced plasminogen, a fetal plasminogen, reduced PAI-1, increased tPA and a fetal fibrinogen) suggest that the regulation of plasmin generation by fibrin and endothelial cell surfaces will differ from adults [22–24]. There are important development differences in the components of the fibrinolytic system between infancy and childhood. In cord blood, during the early postnatal period, the plasma concentrations of plasminogen and α_2AP are decreased to 50 and 80% of adult values, respectively. Furthermore, plasma concentrations of tPA, uPA and PAI-1 are significantly increased in plasma from newborns on day 1 of life compared to adult values. Histidine-rich glycoprotein (HRG), another fibrinolytic inhibitor, retards fibrinolysis by interfering with the ability of plasminogen to bind to fibrin. It has been observed that newborns have significantly lower plasminogen and HRG levels when compared with those of adults [25]. In another study, plasminogen isolated from 60 full-term newborns differed from adult plasminogen in carbohydrate composition, kinetic activation constants, and cell binding [26]. Differences in all these parameters suggested a basis for the decreased fibrinolytic activity observed in neonates. Indeed, Andrew et al. [27] has shown that the ratio of tPA/PAI-1 is reversed throughout childhood, suggesting that the fibrinolytic system is suppressed compared to adults. In order to determine mechanisms involved in developmental differences during fibrinolysis, the formation and fate of plasmin must be assessed as moderated by physiological surfaces.

It has been well recognized that lipoprotein (a) [Lp(a)] is a complex lipoprotein particle that contains a cholesterol-rich, low density lipoprotein (LDL)-like moiety and a specific, carbohydrate-rich protein, apo(a), linked by covalent and noncovalent forces to apo B-100 of LDL [28]. Apo(a) is a highly polymorphic protein with a large degree of structural homology with the coagulation proenzyme plasminogen. Due to its structural homology to both LDL and plasminogen, Lp(a) can potentially be involved in both the pathophysiological process of atherosclerosis and thrombosis in human coronoary artery disease [29]. Therefore, there is evidence that apo(a) can interfere with the fibrinolytic system. Thus Lp(a) is an important issue affecting the mechanism of plasmin activity. In the present study, components of the fibrinolytic system were measured during in vitro plasmin generation in adult or cord plasma in the presence of fibrin monomer.

Design and Methods

Specimen Collection

In vitro plasmin generation was assessed in venous plasma from umbilical cords and adults on plastic surfaces in the presence of fibrin monomer. Umbilical cord blood was obtained immediately after delivery by withdrawing venous blood from double-clamped umbilical cords into 3.2% Na_3-citrate (volume of blood:volume of citrate = 9:1), followed by centrifugation at 3,000 *g* for 20 min at 4°C to obtain supernatant plasma. All plasmas were from uneventful, full-term deliveries (37–41 weeks' gestational age) with appropriate birth weight and Apgar scores. Cord plasmas from 20 cords were pooled for experiments. Normal adult pool plasma was from Cryocheck No. 1830.

Materials

Chromogenic substrate S-2251 was purchased from Dia Pharma (West Chester, Ohio, USA). Desafib, tPA, and plasmin-α_2AP (PAP) enzyme-linked immunosorbent assay (ELISA) kits were from American Diagnostica (Greenwich, Conn., USA), while plasminogen and PAI-1 were from Molecular Innovations (Southfield, Mich., USA). Soybean trypsin inhibitor was obtained from Sigma (Oakville, Canada). tPA STOP solution and lipoprotein [Lp(a)] were purchased from Calbiochem (La Jolla, Calif., USA). Plasminogen and PAI ELISA kits were from Affinity Biologicals (Ancaster, Canada). A plate-reading spectrophotometer (Spectra Max Plus, Molecular Devices, Sunnyvale, Calif., USA) was used to detect products in the assays. Sample diluent green and conjugate diluent red were bought from ALerCHEK (Portland, Me., USA). Commercial standards and controls (Dade Behring, Marburg, Germany) were used for α_2AP and plasminogen ELISAs.

Total Plasmin

Plasmin generation was performed using a published method [30] with modifications. The reaction mixture consisted of 200 µl of citrated adult or cord plasma (prewarmed at 37°C) followed by 200 µl of solution (prewarmed at 37°C) containing buffer (0.036 *M* Na acetate, 0.036 *M* Na diethylbarbituric acid, 0.145 *M* NaCl, pH 7.4), tPA (2.5 µg), with or without soluble fibrin complex (2 µl Desafib). The above reaction mixture was placed in microtubes. Timed (0–120 min) subsamples (50 µl) were taken into 450 µl of 0.5 m*M* of S-2251 in buffer containing PAI-1 (0.0625 µg) to stop further plasmin generation. The subsample was incubated for 15 min in substrate and reaction stopped by addition of 50% of acetic acid. The absorbance was measured at a wavelength of 405 nm in the spectrophotometer.

Plasmin Bound to α_2M

The protocol for measurement of plasmin bound to α_2M was the same as that for total plasmin above, but subsamples (50 µl) from the reaction mixture were placed into buffer containing PAI-1 (0.0625 µg) and soybean trypsin inhibitor (50 µg). After 120 min, chromogenic substrate S-2251 was added and, after 15 min incubation, the substrate hydrolysis stopped by the addition of 100 µl of 50% acetic acid. Any residual activity not inhibited by PAI-1 or soybean trypsin inhibitor was from plasmin entrapped within α_2M. In other experiments, similarly timed (0–120 min) subsamples (50 µl) from the above reaction mixture [buffer, plasma, activator (tPA), soluble fibrin (Desafib)] were sampled into 450 µl of the buffer containing PAI-1 (0.0625 µg) + soybean trypsin inhibitor (50 µg). These samples were stored in 100 µl aliquots at –80°C for analysis of plasminogen, α_2AP, PAI-1, and PAP complexes using ELISAs (see below).

PAP Complex Assay

This ELISA employed a murine monoclonal antibody specific against the antigen in the human PAP complex as the capture antibody (American Diagnostica). Plasma samples were incubated in the microtest wells precoated with the antibody, extraneous proteins were washed away, and a horseradish peroxidase (HRP)-conjugated monoclonal antibody directed against a different epitope of the PAP complex was added to complete the formation of an antibody-antigen-antibody 'sandwich'. The addition of a 3,3′,5,5′-tetramethylbenzidine substrate, and its subsequent reaction with HRP allowed for quantitation. Sensitivity was increased by the addition of a sulfuric acid stop solution, yielding a yellow color. Molar concentrations of PAP complex levels were determined by comparing values with those from a standard curve.

Plasminogen Assay

Plasma analyses for plasminogen concentrations were performed by capturing onto a microtiter plate coated with a capture antibody [affinity-purified goat anti-human plasminogen IgG (PG-EIA-C), Amersham Biosciences, Baie d'Urfe, Canada]. After washing the plate to remove unbound proteins, the capture analytes were detected by incubating with another antibody [peroxidase-linked anti-human plasminogen (PF-EIA-D)] conjugated to HRP to react with *o*-phenylenediamine to give a colored end product. After a fixed time, the reaction was stopped and the absorbance of each well in the microtiter plate was determined. As the concentration of the capture antibody and detecting antibody was fixed, the color generated was proportional to the concentration of analytes present. The selectivity of the ELISA antibody for plasminogen was tested by use of the detecting antibody to probe Western blots of plasmin generation time samples.

α_2AP Assay

This assay was done by the use of an affinity-purified goat anti-human α_2AP IgG (GA2AP-AP) as a detecting antibody and a peroxidase-conjugated goat anti-human α_2AP IgG (GA2AP-HRP) as a detecting antibody in an ELISA kit (Affinity Biologicals). The plates were coated with GA2AP-AP at 5 µg/well and incubated overnight at 4°C. After washing, samples and standards were prepared with diluent green and applied 100 µl/well for 60 min at ambient temperature. GA2AP-HRP was applied at 1/1,000 dilution in conjugate diluent red and applied 100 µl/well for 60 min at ambient temperature.

PAI-1 Assay

This ELISA was done by the use of monoclonal antibody MAI-12 (Biopool, Ventura, Calif., USA) for antigen capture, coated at 2 µg/ml, 100 µl/well overnight at 4°C. Samples and standards were diluted in the sample diluent green and applied 100 µl/well for 90 min at ambient temperature. Human PAI-1 was used as standard. Detecting antibody [peroxidase-conjugated sheep anti-human PAI-1 IgG; SAPAI-HRP (Affinity Biologicals)] was diluted 1/1,000 in 'conjugate diluent red' and applied 100 µl/well for 60 min at ambient temperature and detected with *o*-phenylenediamine substrate. Samples were read at 490 nm in a spectrophotometer.

Effect of Add-Back Plasminogen

Plasminogen was added to cord plasma to increase plasminogen concentrations by 1.4, 1.0 and 0.5 U/ml. Plasminogen was added into the cord plasma reaction mixture (containing buffer, tPA and fibrin monomer, Desafib) at the start of the experiment. Plasmin generation experiment was then carried out as mentioned above following the published method [30].

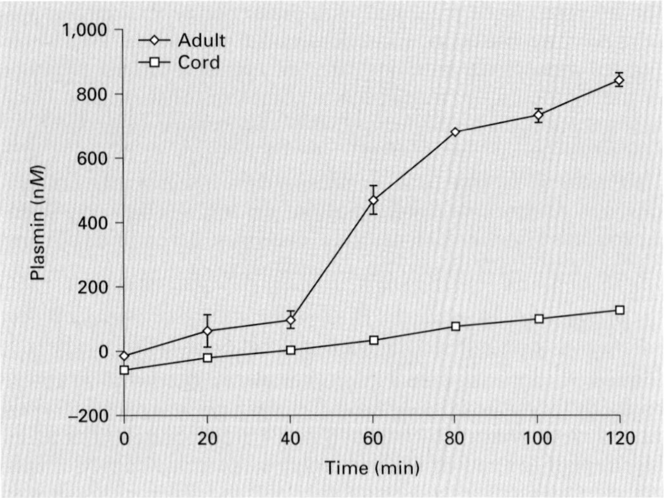

Fig. 1. Total plasmin generation in adult and cord plasmas on plastic surface. Reactions were carried out on plastic in either adult or cord plasmas containing tPA + soluble fibrin complex (Desafib). At various time points, total plasmin activity was determined by subsampling into S-2251 chromogenic substrate + PAI-1 to stop further plasmin generation. Plasma concentrations of plasmin were calculated by reference of activities to a standard curve of purified plasmin reacted with substrate under the same conditions. Results are given as mean ± SE (n ≥ 5).

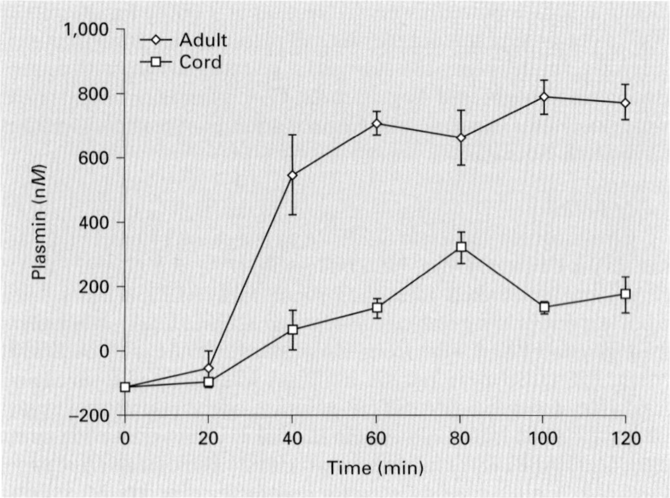

Fig. 2. Total plasmin generation in adult and cord plasmas on endothelial cell surface. Reactions were carried out on HUVEC in either adult or cord plasmas containing tPA + soluble fibrin complex (Desafib). At various time points total plasmin activity was determined by subsampling into S-2251 chromogenic substrate + PAI-1 to stop further plasmin generation. Plasma concentrations of plasmin were calculated by reference of activities to a standard curve of purified plasmin reacted with substrate under the same conditions. Results are given as mean ± SE (n ≥ 5).

Effect of Lp(a)

The effect of Lp(a) on plasmin generation in adult and cord plasma was determined. The Lp(a) was added at concentrations of 0, 0.5, 1.0, and 2.77 mg/ml. Lp(a) was added to reaction mixtures of adult or cord plasmas at the start of experiment. The plasmin generation experiment was then performed as described above.

Statistical Analysis

Data was compared for significant differences using either the Student t test (in the case of two groups) or by analysis of variance (ANOVA, for more than two groups). Upon finding a significant difference within several groups by ANOVA, testing between two groups within that set was carried out by t test. A value of $p < 0.05$ was considered significant and results were expressed as mean ± SE.

Results

Plasmin Generation on Plastic Surfaces

Figure 1 shows total plasmin concentrations in adult and cord pooled plasmas on plastic surfaces. It was observed that total plasmin generated over 2 h in cord plasma was significantly lower ($p < 0.01$) than that in adult plasma. There was significant free plasmin activity generated in experiments with adult plasma, although most plasmin was complexed quickly by α_2M and α_2AP. The onset of plasmin generation in adult plasma occurred by 60 min and showed an exponential increase. In cord plasma, total plasmin activity increased after 80 min, but the amount of plasmin generated was less than 20% of that in adult plasma. The activity of plasmin bound to α_2M at the final end point (120 min) was also measured. Significantly more α_2M was bound to plasmin in adult plasma (714 ± 22 n*M*) compared to that in cord plasma (100 ± 1 n*M*; $p < 0.01$).

Plasmin Generation on Cell Surfaces

The total plasmin generation was also determined on human umbilical vein endothelial cells (HUVEC) (fig. 2). The onset of plasmin generation on endothelial surfaces was earlier (40 min) than on plastic surfaces, regardless of plasma type. In cord plasma, the amount of plasmin generated was also increased compared to that on plastic. Again, however, total plasmin generated was significantly greater in adult plasma compared to cord plasma ($p < 0.05$) up to the final equilibrium point at 2 h.

PAP Complexes

To obtain further insight into the mechanisms responsible for differing plasmin concentrations in cord plasma compared to adult plasma, time samples from the plasmin generation experiments were analyzed for PAP complexes. The PAP complexes showed the same trend as that for total plasmin generation over time (fig. 3). The concentrations of the PAP complexes were significantly lower in cord plasma than in adult plasma at the end of 2 h of plasmin generation. The increase in PAP complex formation in cord plasma diverged from that generated in adult plasma from 20 to 60 min after initiation of plasminogen activation.

Plasminogen

In order to assess the potential to form plasmin in the different plasmas, the amount of plasminogen was measured in time samples from the initiation (0 min) to termination (120 min) of the experiment (fig. 4). The plasminogen concentration at 0 min in adult plasma (1,526 ± 40 n*M*) was significantly higher than that in starting cord plasma (922 ± 62 n*M*; $p < 0.05$). Over the course of the experiments, however, total plasminogen decreased significantly faster in the adult plasma compared to cord plasma ($p < 0.05$). In fact, from 80 to 120 min of plasmin generation, differences in plasminogen concentrations between adult and cord plasmas had largely disappeared. Over the 2-hour time course, the consumption of plasminogen in adult plasma was 51% and 72% in the case of cord plasma, which was calculated on the basis of initial and final values of plasminogen.

α_2AP and PAI-1 Consumption

In order to assess if there were any differences in capacity to inhibit plasmin as it was generated, α_2AP inhibitor levels were determined. The concentration of α_2AP in the adult and cord plasmas over the course of 2 h is shown in figure 5. As expected, starting adult plasma levels (902 ± 26 n*M*) were significantly higher than those of cord plasma (731 ± 50.2 n*M*; $p < 0.05$). Over the time course, significantly more α_2AP was consumed in adult compared to cord plasma, which is consistent with inhibition of the generated plasmin from increased amount of activated plasminogen in adult plasma (fig. 4). However, both adult and cord plasma concentrations of α_2AP dropped until they reached similar plateaus from 60 to 120 min with significant amounts of inhibitor remaining (646 ± 42 n*M* in adult plasma and 607 ± 24 n*M* in cord plasma).

To assess any differences in the inhibition of plasminogen activator, PAI-1 levels were measured in adult and cord plasmas in the time samples (fig. 6). Again, initial adult plasma concentrations of PAI-1 (2.43 ± 0.1 n*M*) were higher compared to those in cord plasma (1.5 ± 0.017 n*M*). Nevertheless, levels of adult (1.9 ± 0.15 n*M*)

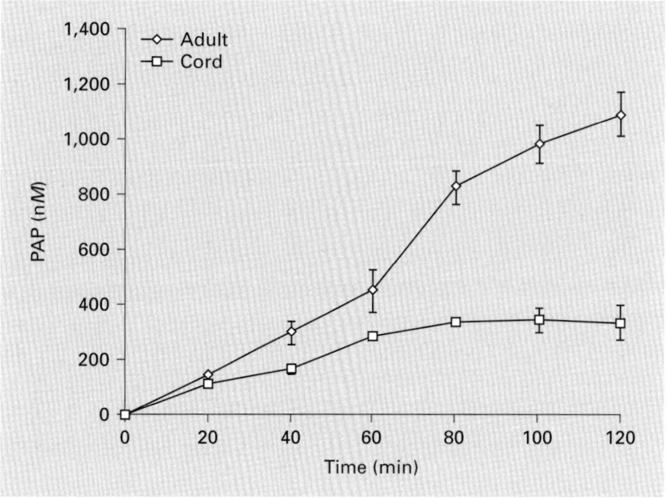

Fig. 3. PAP complexes in adult and cord plasmas on plastic. Reactions were carried out on plastic in either adult or cord plasmas containing tPA + soluble fibrin complex (Desafib). PAP complexes were determined by ELISA in time samples of the reaction mixture taken into PAI-1 + soybean trypsin inhibitor to stop further PAP complex generation. Results are given as mean ± SE ($n \geq 5$).

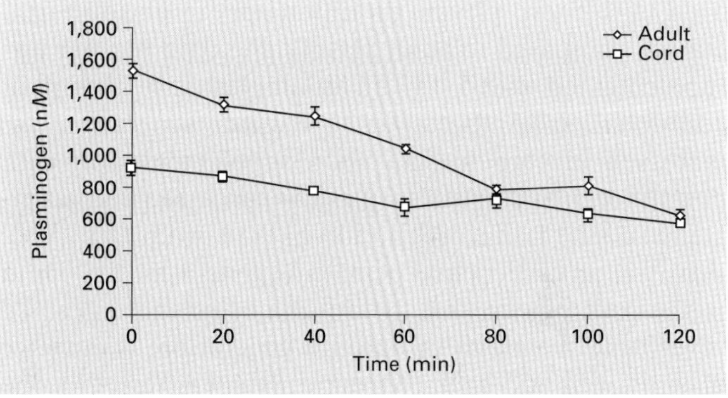

Fig. 4. Plasminogen consumption in adult and cord plasmas during plasmin generation on plastic. Reactions were carried out on plastic in either adult or cord plasmas containing tPA + soluble fibrin complex (Desafib). Plasminogen was measured by ELISA in time samples of the reaction mixture taken into PAI-1 + soybean trypsin inhibitor to stop further plasmin generation. Results are given as mean ± SE ($n \geq 5$).

and cord plasma (1.59 ± 0.045 n*M*) were not significantly different ($p > 0.2$) after 2 h of plasmin generation and only minor proportions of the inhibitor were consumed.

Effect of Add-Back Plasminogen

It is well known that the cord plasma has low plasminogen concentrations. To determine the effect of plasmin-

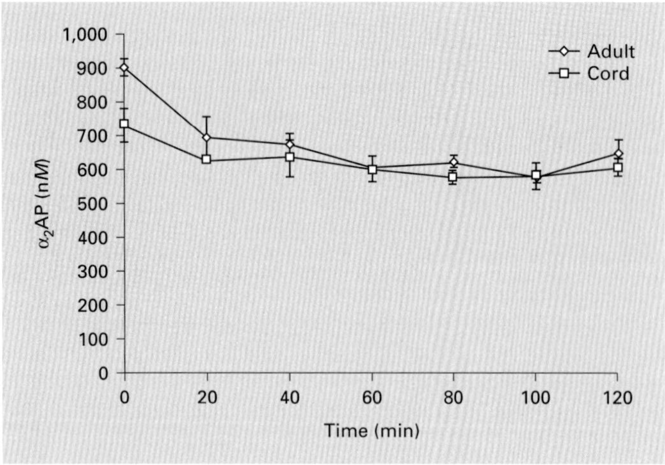

Fig. 5. α_2AP in adult and cord plasmas during plasmin generation on plastic. Reactions were carried out on plastic in either adult or cord plasmas containing tPA + soluble fibrin complex (Desafib). α_2AP was measured by ELISA in time samples of the reaction mixture taken into PAI-1 + soybean trypsin inhibitor to stop further plasmin formation and inhibition. Results are given as mean ± SE (n ≥ 5).

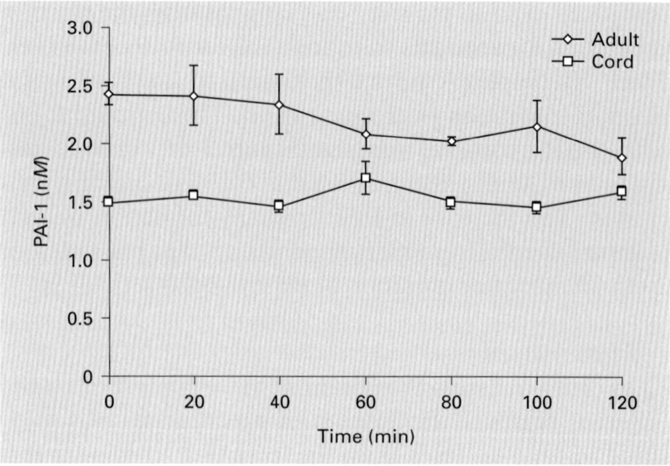

Fig. 6. PAI-1 in adult and cord plasmas during plasmin generation on plastic. Reactions were carried out on plastic in either adult or cord plasmas containing tPA + soluble fibrin complex (Desafib). PAI-1 was measured by ELISA in time samples of the reaction mixture taken into soybean trypsin inhibitor to stop further plasmin formation and inhibition. Results are given as mean ± SE (n ≥ 5).

ogen in the cord plasma on differences in plasmin generation compared to adult plasma, the cord plasma was supplemented with 1.4 U/ml (adult plasma = 1 U/ml) of additional plasminogen (fig. 7). Plasmin generation was increased in cord plasma upon supplementation with plasminogen and final total plasmin surpassed that generated in adult plasma with no add-back plasminogen. Also, there was an earlier onset of plasmin generation at 20 min in the cord plasma due to addition of plasminogen. To investigate the trend in plasmin generation, a range of plasminogen add-back concentrations was tested in the cord plasma. Results for total plasmin generation in cord plasmas supplemented with additional plasminogen concentrations of 0.5 and 1.0 U/ml were compared with non-supplemented cord plasma (fig. 8). Plasmin generation was increased 6-fold after the addition of 0.5 U/ml of plasminogen (648 ± 26.6 n*M*) relative to cord plasma with no supplementation (127 ± 0.12 n*M*). The addition of 1.0 U/ml of plasminogen showed a further increase in plasmin generation (1,003 ± 26.4 n*M*).

Effect of Lp(a)

Plasmin generation was significantly inhibited in adult plasma upon addition of 0.5 mg Lp(a)/ml (fig. 9). When cord plasma was supplemented with Lp(a) (0.5 mg/ml), no inhibitory effect was observed. The effect of Lp(a) was further tested on plasmin generation in adult plasma at higher concentrations (0.5, 1.0 and 2.77 mg/ml; fig. 10). The effect on plasmin generation was inhibitory for all concentrations tested in the adult plasma.

Discussion

The hemostatic system in newborns, infants and children differs from adults. The age-dependent, physiological differences of the fibrinolytic system in the young (reduced plasminogen, a fetal plasminogen, reduced PAI-1, increased tPA and a fetal fibrinogen) suggest that the regulation of plasmin generation by fibrin and/or an endothelial surfaces will differ from adults [22, 23, 31]. However, whether age-related variation in fibrinolysis is due to increased plasmin generation or overcoming plasmin inhibition (to verify the mechanism) has not previously been studied. Also, the effects of cells or Lp(a) on these parameters were not investigated earlier. Therefore, the present work completes a broad mechanistic investigation of all parameters associated with the fibrinolytic system in adults and newborns.

The fibrinolytic data in this study shows that plasminogen activation by tPA was much faster in adults than newborns under physiological conditions in vitro (fig. 1). The generation of plasmin was increased in adult plasma as compared to cord plasma up to a final equilibrium con-

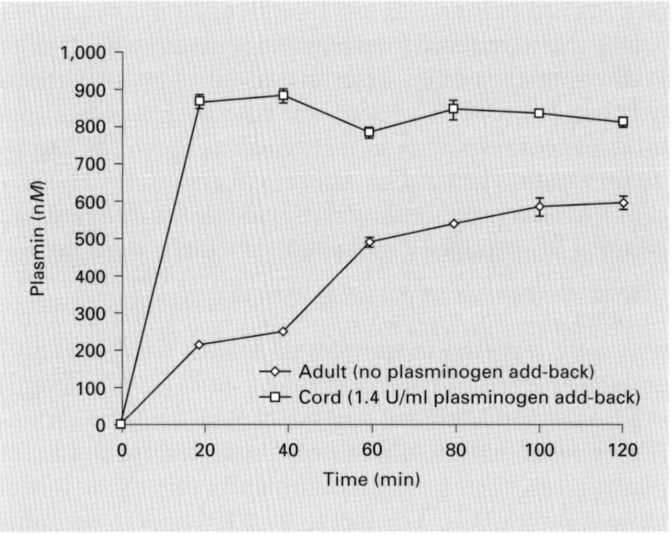

Fig. 7. Comparison of total plasmin generation in adult plasma or cord plasma with added plasminogen. Reactions [tPA + soluble fibrin monomer (Desafib)] were carried out on plastic in either adult plasma or cord plasma supplemented with 1.4 U/ml of plasminogen. At various time points, total plasmin activity was determined by subsampling into S-2251 chromogenic substrate + PAI-1 to stop further plasmin generation. Plasma concentrations of plasmin were calculated by reference of activities to a standard curve of purified plasmin reacted with substrate under the same conditions. Results are given as mean ± SE (n ≥ 5).

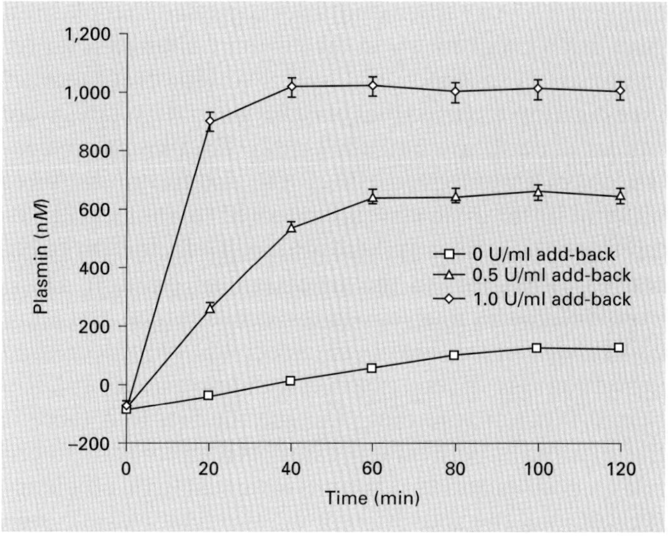

Fig. 8. Total plasmin generation in cord plasma supplemented with varying amounts of plasminogen. Reactions [with tPA + soluble fibrin monomer (Desafib)] were carried out on plastic in cord plasma supplemented with varying amounts of plasminogen. At various time points, total plasmin activity was determined by subsampling into S-2251 chromogenic substrate + PAI-1 to stop further plasmin generation. Plasma concentrations of plasmin were calculated by reference of activities to a standard curve of purified plasmin reacted with substrate under the same conditions. Results are given as mean ± SE (n ≥ 5).

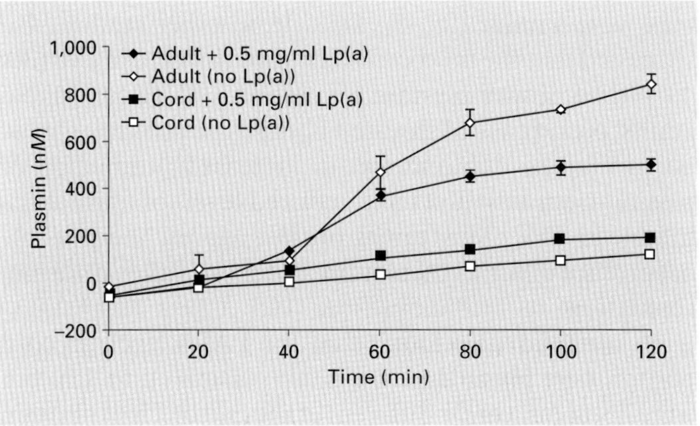

Fig. 9. Total plasmin generation in adult and cord plasmas in the presence of Lp(a). Reactions [with tPA + soluble fibrin complex (Desafib)] were carried out on plastic in either adult or cord plasmas containing added Lp(a). At various time points, total plasmin activity was determined by subsampling into S-2251 chromogenic substrate + PAI-1 to stop further plasmin generation. Plasma concentrations of plasmin were calculated by reference of activities to a standard curve of purified plasmin reacted with substrate under the same conditions. Results are given as mean ± SE (n ≥ 5).

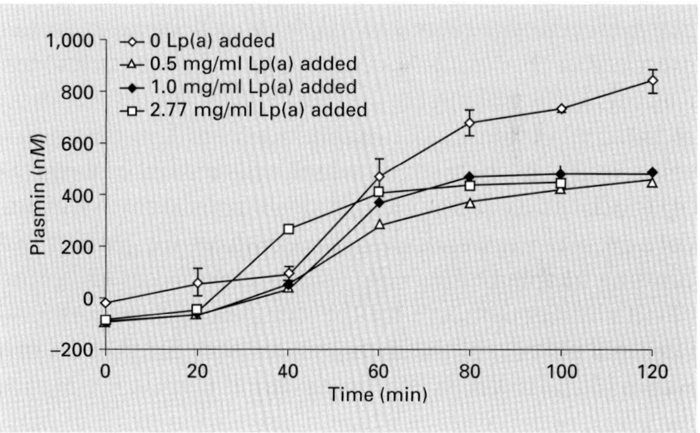

Fig. 10. Total plasmin generation in adult plasma supplemented with varying amounts of Lp(a). Reactions [with tPA + soluble fibrin complex (Desafib)] were carried out on plastic in adult plasma containing varying amounts of added Lp(a). At various time points, total plasmin activity was determined by subsampling into S-2251 chromogenic substrate + PAI-1 to stop further plasmin generation. Plasma concentrations of plasmin were calculated by reference of activities to a standard curve of purified plasmin reacted with substrate under the same conditions. Results are given as mean ± SE (n ≥ 5).

dition at 2 h. An earlier study [30] suggested that plasmin generation experiments in the newborn showed a slower response to exogenous uPA and tPA. However, another investigation reported that plasmin generation rates were similar in newborns and adults [32]. The plasma concentrations of plasminogen, tPA, PAI-1 and the inhibitors of plasmin differ in newborns compared to adults [22]. Altered concentrations of these fibrinolytic factors probably caused differences in the generation of plasmin. However, differences in glycosylation between fetal and adult plasminogen have also been associated with decreased activation rate of fetal plasminogen to plasmin [26]. Reported functional findings include the fact that there is less binding of both fetal plasminogen glycoforms to cellular receptors and that there is lower catalytic efficiency ($kcat/K_m$) of the activation of the two fetal plasminogen types by tPA [33]. Binding of plasmin to α_2M provided a significant portion of the plasmin inhibition, especially in the case of cord plasma. This outcome is not surprising, given that it is well known that the plasma concentration of α_2M is significantly increased at birth [22].

On endothelial surfaces, plasmin generation occurred earlier and was increased in both adult and cord plasmas (fig. 2) compared to corresponding results on plastic surfaces. In agreement with our findings, previous studies showed that binding of plasminogen [20, 34], tPA [35], or uPA [21] to endothelial surfaces accelerated plasmin generation. Another report has suggested that when Glu-plasminogen was bound to HUVEC cell surfaces in the presence of tPA or uPA, conversion to Lys-plasminogen was markedly enhanced, suggesting that the stimulation of the conversion of Glu-plasminogen to Lys-plasminogen is a key mechanism by which cells enhance plasminogen activation [36]. This study is consistent with our data on increased endothelial-based plasmin generation. Binding of tPA to HUVEC occurs at two sites [37], one of which may compete for the same sequence on the N-terminal portion of the B chain necessary for PAI-1 inhibition [35]. However, our results are the first to compare the effect of cell surface plasmin generation in adult plasma with that of cord plasma.

It has been shown that the most important inhibitor of plasmin is α_2AP. Plasmin reacts with α_2AP to form a 1:1 stoichiometric complex (PAP) that has no further enzymatic activity. Higher PAP complex formation in adult compared to cord plasma (fig. 3) suggested that the potential for free plasmin generation from plasminogen was reduced in cord plasma (fig. 4). Since PAP complex levels increased over time, the free plasmin generated was complexed quickly by α_2AP. The concentration of PAP complex in cord plasma was less than in adult plasma, as expected due to reduced total plasmin generated (fig. 1). The PAP complex is often described as an index of fibrinolytic activity [38]. However, our data indicates that this inhibitor complex may in fact reflect as much the capacity for plasmin generation as fibrin degradation. The level of PAP has been measured previously for different age groups [39]. Analyses indicated that there were no significant differences among all age groups (1 year to adults). In other studies, markedly elevated levels of PAP complex were reported in samples of healthy newborns [40] and lower levels of PAP in amniotic fluid [41]. In another study, detailed kinetic analysis of PAP complex formation showed that the differences between fetal and adult plasmin reactions were predominantly due to the initial loose complex [42]. The fact that differences in the inhibition kinetics between neonates and adults could only be obtained in the absence or at low levels of tranexamic acid suggests that these differences are dependent on kringle structures. It could, therefore, be that differences in glycosylation may account for the functional differences in PAP formation [42].

Concentrations of α_2AP decreased over time in both adult and cord plasma (fig. 5), in correspondence to the time-dependent increase in PAP complex levels. Since α_2AP is present in excess relative to potential plasmin generated in vivo, little free plasmin would be expected to circulate. Final levels of α_2AP in adult and cord plasmas were similar (fig. 5). Data from other studies also suggested that the newborn has normal levels of α_2AP [30, 43, 44] but slower plasmin generation [30]. In contrast to adults, occurrence of elevated fibrinolytic activity in newborns may be due, mainly, to increased production of plasminogen activators and reduced levels of fibrinolysis inhibitors [45]. This might protect against the possible occurrence of intravascular fibrin deposits after placental separation.

In our study, we found that the PAI-1 levels in cord plasma were lower than the adult plasma up to 1 h, but were not significantly different at the end of 2 h of plasmin generation (fig. 6). Our findings of decreased PAI-1 levels in cord plasma confirm other data showing that plasma concentrations of PAI-1 measured in cord plasma are different than those measured in cord plasma at 1 day of life [46, 47]. Taking into account comparison of PAI-1 in cord plasma to that in day 1 plasma, the present study has attempted to quantitate the likely relative impact of plasma from a developmental stage on plasmin generation. Since obtaining day 1 plasma was extremely difficult, our results may be more representative of activities at birth. Previous work [48] showed that lower levels of von Willebrand factor and PAI, and higher levels of D-dimer were found in newborns as compared to their mothers.

We also determined the plasminogen consumption in adult and cord plasma during the period of plasmin generation. Data from plasminogen analyses inferred that a possible cause of very low plasmin generation in cord plasma might be due to reduced starting plasminogen antigen levels (fig. 4). Numerous investigators have already reported that cord plasma contains 50% of the plasminogen activity and protein levels of adult plasma [22, 49–53]. Whether a functional abnormality exists in newborn plasminogen is unclear. It is known that the plasminogen level decreases in full-term newborns [50]. In our study, total consumption of plasminogen was found to be 51% for adult and 72% for cord plasma during plasmin generation.

When cord plasma was supplemented with higher concentrations of plasminogen, the decreased plasmin generation, relative to adult plasma, was overcome (fig. 7, 8). When the concentration of the plasminogen supplementation in the cord plasma was equal to adult, the amount of plasmin generated was similar to adult levels. Results of our study strongly support the fact that the plasminogen concentration is the critical feature responsible for decreased fibrinolysis in cord plasma. Thus, our data was compatible with the conclusions of others [30, 51] that lower plasminogen concentrations in cord plasma give reduced plasmin generation with respect to that in adult plasma.

It has been hypothesized earlier that elevated Lp(a) levels lead to decreased fibrinolysis, due to the close structural homology with plasminogen [52]. Although the mechanism of action of Lp(a) is not fully understood, there is evidence that apo Lp(a) can interfere with the fibrinolytic system [53, 54]. Since Lp(a) cannot be converted into a plasmin-like enzyme, it may cause an inhibition of plasminogen activation by competing with plasminogen for lysine binding sites. Our results showed consistency with earlier reports that Lp(a) has an inhibitory effect on the adult plasma fibrinolysis. However, in cord plasma, Lp(a) had no antagonistic effects on plasmin generation (fig. 9). Early in vitro studies on the impact of Lp(a) on tPA-mediated plasminogen activation suggested an inhibitory effect of Lp(a) on this process by competition of plasminogen for tPA [54]. Thus, lower plasminogen concentrations in cord plasma or altered affinity of newborn plasminogen for fibrin or tPA may be factors in the relative differences in apo Lp(a) on plasmin generation in cord versus adult plasma.

To our knowledge, no previous work has been done to test the effect of lipoprotein on plasminogen activation in cord plasma. However, it has been shown that in subjects heterozygous for the apo Lp(a) trait, the influence of the various apo Lp(a) isoforms on fibrinolysis depends on their affinity for fibrin and on their concentrations relative to each other and to plasminogen [55]. According to these data, high levels of Lp(a) and low plasminogen concentrations are conditions that promote the deleterious effect of Lp(a) in a majority of nephrotic children [55]. Correspondingly, the difference in Lp(a) effect on plasmin generation in cord plasma may have more to do with structural variation in plasminogen between newborns and adults.

Dose response of lipoprotein on plasmin was studied in adult plasma (fig. 10). Concentrations of Lp(a), up to 2.77 mg/ml, displayed a similar antifibrinolytic activity. It has been observed recently that Lp(a) isoform size is inversely correlated with plasma Lp(a) levels [29]. Furthermore, Lp(a) levels in plasma are strongly correlated to the rate of plasmin formation and support the hypothesis that high Lp(a) is directly involved in reducing plasmin activity [29]. Using relatively concentrated amounts of Lp(a) in our experiments (0.5–3 mg/ml) a plateau effect on plasmin generation inhibition was observed.

In conclusion, our study shows that plasmin generation induced by tPA in vitro is reduced in newborn compared to adult plasma. Decreased amounts of plasminogen were consumed in cord plasma that is coincident with the diminished plasmin and PAP complex generated in newborn relative to adult plasma. The addition of plasminogen in cord plasma increased plasmin generation. Thus, we speculate that the ability to eliminate thrombi in newborns is reduced due to decreased capacity to generate plasmin. Decreased plasmin generation in cord plasma is likely due to decreased plasminogen concentration rather than increased inhibition. Studies are underway to further illuminate the mechanisms related to the suppression of the fibrinolytic system of newborns in vivo.

Acknowledgements

This work was supported by a grant from the Heart and Stroke Foundation of Ontario (No. NA5639). Anthony Chan holds a Research Scholarship award from the Heart and Stroke Foundation of Canada. During the course of this study, Dr. Maureen Andrew passed away. She was instrumental in the initiation of this work and inspired its direction. We dedicate this paper to her memory.

References

1 Mackinnon S, Walker ID, Davidson JF, Walker JJ: Plasma fibrinolysis during and after normal childbirth. Br J Haematol 1987;65:339–342.
2 Andrew M: Developmental hemostasis: relevance to hemostatic problems during childhood. Semin Thromb Hemost 1995;21:341–356.
3 Pinacho A: Paramo JA, Ezcurdia M, Rocha E: Evaluation of the fibrinolytic system in full-term neonates. Int J Clin Lab Res 1995;25: 149–152.
4 Christensen U, Sottrup-Jensen L: Mechanism of alpha 2-macroglobulin-proteinase interactions. Biochemistry 1984;23:6619–6626.
5 Wiman B, Wallen P: The specific interaction between plasminogen and fibrin. Thromb Res 1977;10:213–222.
6 Wallen P, Wiman B: Characterization of human plasminogen. I. On the relationship between different molecular forms of plasminogen demonstrated in plasma and found in purified preparations. Biochim Biophys Acta 1970;221:20–30.
7 Dhainaut JF, Yan SB, Cariou A, Mira JP: Soluble thrombomodulin, plasma-derived unactivated protein C, and recombinant human activated protein C in sepsis. Crit Care Med 2002;30:S318–S324.
8 Rezaie AR: Vitronectin functions as a cofactor for rapid inhibition of activated protein C by plasminogen activator inhibitor-1. Implications for the mechanism of profibrinolytic action of activated protein C. J Biol Chem 2001; 276:15567–15570.
9 Sakamoto T, Ogawa H, Takazoe K, Yoshimura M, Shimomura H, Moriyama Y, Arai H, Okajima K: Effect of activated protein C on plasma plasminogen activator inhibitor activity in patients with acute myocardial infarction treated with alteplase: comparison with unfractionated heparin. J Am Coll Cardiol 2003; 42:1389–1394.
10 Wun TC, Capuano A: Initiation and regulation of fibrinolysis in human plasma at the plasminogen activator level. Blood 1987;69:1354–1362.
11 Collen D: On the regulation and control of fibrinolysis. Thromb Haemost 1980;43:77–89.
12 Collen D, Lijnen HR: Basic and clinical aspects of fibrinolysis and thrombolysis. Blood 1991;78:3114–3124.
13 Marin ML, Veith FJ, Cynamon J, Sanchez LA, Lyon RT, Levine BA, Bakal CW, Suggs WD, Wengerter KR, Rivers SP: Initial experience with transluminally placed endovascular grafts for the treatment of complex vascular lesions. Ann Surg 1995;222:449–465.
14 Booth NA: Fibrinolysis and thrombosis. Baillières Best Pract Res Clin Haematol 1999;12: 423–433.
15 Mosesson MW: Fibrinogen and fibrin polymerization: appraisal of the binding events. Blood Coagul Fibrinolysis 1997;8:257–267.
16 Smokovitis A: Regions of constantly increased plasminogen activator activity along the intima of the normal aorta. Haemostasis 1978;7: 303–319.
17 Mishima A, Asano M, Saito T, Yamamoto S, Ukai T, Yoshitomi H, Matsumoto K, Manabe T: Pulmonary blood flow regulates plasma tissue plasminogen activator concentrations in patients with congenital heart defects. J Thorac Cardiovasc Surg 1997;113:742–747.
18 Van Hinsberg VW, Sprengers ED, Kooistra T: Effect of thrombin on the production of plasminogen activators and PA inhibitor-1 by human foreskin microvascular endothelial cells. Thromb Haemost 1987;57:148–153.
19 Reininger AJ, Heinzmann U, Reininger CB, Friedrich P, Wurzinger LJ: Flow mediated fibrin thrombus formation in an endothelium-lined model. Thromb Res 1994;74:629–641.
20 Christiansen VJ, Sims PJ, Hamilton KK: Complement C5b-9 increases plasminogen binding and activation on human endothelial cells. Arterioscler Thromb Vasc Biol 1997;17: 164–171.
21 Fan Z, Larson PJ, Bognacki J, Raghunath PN, Tomaszewski JE, Kuo A, Canziani G, Chaiken I, Cines DB, Higazi AA: Tissue factor regulates plasminogen binding and activation. Blood 1998;91:1987–1998.
22 Andrew M, Paes B, Milner R, Johnston M, Mitchell L, Tollefsen DM, Powers P: Development of the human coagulation system in the full-term infant. Blood 1987;70:165–172.
23 Andrew M, Mitchell L, Berry LR, Schmidt B, Hatton MW: Fibrinogen has a rapid turnover in the healthy newborn lamb. Pediatr Res 1988;23:249–252.
24 Ries M: Molecular and functional properties of fetal plasminogen and its possible influence on clot lysis in the neonatal period. Semin Thromb Hemost 1997;23:247–252.
25 Corrigan JJ Jr, Jeter M: Histidine-rich glycoprotein and plasminogen plasma levels in term and preterm newborns. Am J Dis Child 1990; 144:825–828.
26 Edelberg JM, Enghild JJ, Pizzo SV, Gonzalez-Gronow M: Neonatal plasminogen displays altered cell surface binding and activation kinetics. Correlation with increased glycosylation of the protein. J Clin Invest 1990;86:107–112.
27 Andrew M, Michelson AD, Bovill E, Leaker M, Massicotte MP: Guidelines for antithrombotic therapy in pediatric patients. J Pediatr 1998; 132:575–588.
28 Testa R, Marcovina SM: The rate of plasmin formation after in vitro clotting is inversely related to lipoprotein(a) plasma levels. Int J Clin Lab Res 1999;29:128–132.
29 Marcovina SM, Koschinsky ML: Evaluation of lipoprotein(a) as a prothrombotic factor: progress from bench to bedside. Curr Opin Lipidol 2003;14:361–366.
30 Corrigan JJ Jr, Sleeth JJ, Jeter M, Lox CD: Newborn's fibrinolytic mechanism: components and plasmin generation. Am J Hematol 1989;32:273–278.
31 Ries M: Molecular and functional properties of fetal plasminogen and its possible influence on clot lysis in the neonatal period. Semin Thromb Hemost 1997;23:247–252.
32 Hilali MM, Gilliver BE: Physiological activation of plasminogen in full term newborn infants. J Clin Pathol 1984;37:1264–1267.
33 Edelberg JM, Enghild JJ, Pizzo SV, Gonzalez-Gronow M: Neonatal plasminogen displays altered cell surface binding and activation kinetics. Correlation with increased glycosylation of the protein. J Clin Invest 1990;86:107–112.
34 Ranson M, Andronicos NM: Plasminogen binding and cancer: promises and pitfalls. Front Biosci 2003;8:S294–S304.
35 Cheng XF, Brohlin M, Pohl G, Back O, Wallen P: Binding of tissue plasminogen activator to endothelial cells. Thromb Res 1995;77:149–164.
36 Gong Y, Kim SO, Felez J, Grella DK, Castellino FJ, Miles LA: Conversion of Glu-plasminogen to Lys-plasminogen is necessary for optimal stimulation of plasminogen activation on the endothelial cell surface. J Biol Chem 2001; 276:19078–19083.
37 Hajjar KA: Assembly of plasmin-generating proteins on the surface of human endothelial cells. Ann Epidemiol 1992;2:419–426.
38 Wiman B, Collen D: On the mechanism of the reaction between human alpha 2-antiplasmin and plasmin. J Biol Chem 1979;254:9291–9297.
39 Montes R, Paramo JA, Angles-Cano E, Rocha E: Development and clinical application of a new ELISA assay to determine plasmin-alpha2-antiplasmin complexes in plasma. Br J Haematol 1996;92:979–985.
40 Knofler R, Hofmann S, Weissbach G, Kuhlisch E, Neef B, Otte M, Pargac N, Nachtrodt G: Molecular markers of the endothelium, the coagulation and the fibrinolytic systems in healthy newborns. Semin Thromb Hemost 1998;24:453–461.
41 Uszynski M, Klyszejko A, Zekanowska E: Plasminogen, alpha(2)-antiplasmin and complexes of plasmin-alpha(2)-antiplasmin (PAP) in amniotic fluid and blood plasma of parturient women. Eur J Obstet Gynecol Reprod Biol 2000;93:167–171.
42 Ries M, Easton RL, Longstaff C, Zenker M, Morris HR, Dell A, Gaffney PJ: Differences between neonates and adults in carbohydrate sequences and reaction kinetics of plasmin and alpha(2)-antiplasmin. Thromb Res 2002;105: 247–256.
43 Andrew M, Vegh P, Johnston M, Bowker J, Ofosu F, Mitchell L: Maturation of the hemostatic system during childhood. Blood 1992; 80:1998–2005.

44 Suarez CR, Walenga J, Mangogna LC, Fareed J: Neonatal and maternal fibrinolysis: activation at time of birth. Am J Hematol 1985;19:365–372.

45 Foley ME, Clayton JK, McNicol GP: Haemostatic mechanisms in maternal, umbilical vein and umbilical artery blood at the time of delivery. Br J Obstet Gynaecol 1977;84:81–87.

46 Astedt B, Lindoff C: Plasminogen activators and plasminogen activator inhibitors in plasma of premature and term newborns. Acta Paediatr 1997;86:111–113.

47 Andrew M, Paes B, Johnston M: Development of the hemostatic system in the neonate and young infant. Am J Pediatr Hematol Oncol 1990;12:95–104.

48 Schneider DM, von Tempelhoff GF, Herrle B, Heilmann L: Maternal and cord blood hemostasis at delivery. J Perinat Med 1997;25:55–61.

49 Ambrus CM, Ambrus JL, Choi TS, Jung O, Mirand EA, Bartfay-Szabo A: The fibrinolysis system and its relationship to disease in the newborn. Am J Pediatr Hematol Oncol 1979;1:251–260.

50 Ekelund H, Finnstrom O: The fibrinolytic system in infants of low birth weight and-or short gestational period. Acta Paediatr Scand Suppl 1970;206(suppl):31.

51 Andrew M, Paes B, Milner R, Johnston M, Mitchell L, Tollefsen DM, Castle V, Powers P: Development of the human coagulation system in the healthy premature infant. Blood 1988;72:1651–1657.

52 Hancock MA, Boffa MB, Marcovina SM, Nesheim ME, Koschinsky ML: Inhibition of plasminogen activation by lipoprotein(a): critical domains in apolipoprotein(a) and mechanism of inhibition on fibrin and degraded fibrin surfaces. J Biol Chem 2003;278:23260–23269.

53 Rouy D, Grailhe P, Nigon F, Chapman J, Angles-Cano E: Lipoprotein(a) impairs generation of plasmin by fibrin-bound tissue-type plasminogen activator. In vitro studies in a plasma milieu. Arterioscler Thromb 1991;11:629–638.

54 Loscalzo J, Weinfeld M, Fless GM, Scanu AM: Lipoprotein(a), fibrin binding, and plasminogen activation. Arteriosclerosis 1990;10:240–245.

55 Hervio L, Durlach V, Girard-Globa A, Angles-Cano E: Multiple binding with identical linkage: a mechanism that explains the effect of lipoprotein(a) on fibrinolysis. Biochemistry 1995;34:13353–13358.

Acta Hæmatologica

Acta Haematol 2006;115:152–156
DOI: 10.1159/000090928

Platelet Function of Newborns as Tested by Cone and Plate(let) Analyzer Correlates with Gestational Age

Y. Levy-Shraga[a] A. Maayan-Metzger[b] A. Lubetsky[c] B. Shenkman[c] J. Kuint[b] U. Martinowitz[c] G. Kenet[c]

[a]Pediatric Department and [b]Department of Neonatology, The Edmond and Lily Safra Children's Hospital and [c]Pediatric Coagulation Service, National Hemophilia Center and Institute of Thrombosis and Hemostasis, Sheba Medical Center, Tel Hashomer and Sackler Faculty of Medicine, Tel Aviv University, Tel Hashomer, Israel

Key Words

Cone and plate(let) analyzer · Platelet function

Abstract

The issue of platelet function in infants and neonates is of interest, and current data are debatable. A new method for assessing platelet function involves using the cone and plate(let) analyzer (CPA), applicable for small (0.2 ml) whole blood volumes. We used polystyrene surface-coated plates to evaluate cord blood neonatal platelet function under flow. One hundred and sixty full-term and 29 preterm infants born at the Sheba Medical Center between March 2003 and January 2004 were evaluated for platelet adhesion measured as surface coverage (SC; the percentage of total area covered by platelets) and platelet aggregation, defined as the average size (AS) of the aggregates. Platelets from preterm infants displayed less platelet adhesion than did those from full-term infants. Platelet SC correlated with gestational age in all infants ($p < 0.05$), and both groups exhibited similar aggregation (AS). AS values, however, were significantly lower than the normal adult range in our laboratory. Infants born to mothers with pregnancy-induced hypertension displayed significantly lower SC. No association was found between CPA and postnatal complications. *Conclusion:* CPA provides a rapid, feasible option for testing platelet function in neonates. Its potential predictive value deserves further attention, and more extensive studies are warranted.

Introduction

Over the past century, the discovery of individual components of the hemostatic system and their interactions has been accompanied by the realization that hemostasis is a dynamic, evolving process that begins in utero [1]. Recent studies have provided reference ranges that delineate age-dependent features of coagulation factors and proteins [2, 3]. Whereas tables of age-related normal values for the levels of coagulation factors facilitate evaluation of infants with secondary hemostasis defects, evaluation of primary hemostatic defects during the neonatal period deserves further attention. Platelet number and volume are similar in neonates as compared to adult values [4–6]. Nevertheless, platelet function testing in the neonatal period is troublesome and requires special consideration. Standard platelet aggregation tests or studies of platelets derived from cord blood using monoclonal antibodies and flow cytometry techniques generally re-

KARGER

Fax +41 61 306 12 34
E-Mail karger@karger.ch
www.karger.com

Accessible online at:
www.karger.com/aha

Gili Kenet, MD
Pediatric Coagulation Service, National Hemophilia Center and
Institute of Thrombosis and Hemostasis, Sheba Medical Center
Tel Hashomer, 52621 (Israel)
Tel. +972 3 530 2120, Fax +972 3 535 1806, E-Mail gili.kenet@sheba.health.gov.il

port the hyporesponsiveness of neonatal platelets [7–11]. The duration of platelet hyporeactivity and its clinical significance, however, have not yet been completely elucidated [11].

One of the methods for assessing platelet function is by using the cone and plate(let) analyzer (CPA). This is a new method for examining platelet adhesion and aggregation on extracellular matrix (ECM) under flow conditions. The method has been used in various platelet disorders, including in infants [12–17]. The use of CPA to evaluate platelet function of neonates has previously been reported [17] in a study applying CPA either to neonatal cord blood samples or neonatal venous blood. Neonatal platelet function test results were similar regardless of blood sampling technique. The potential interpretation of platelet function using very small amounts of venous blood or cord blood makes CPA testing an attractive mode for rapid, feasible evaluation of platelet function in neonates and a candidate test that may be applied for detecting bleeding tendency in neonates [18, 19].

In our prospective single-center study, we aimed at evaluating platelet function of full-term and preterm neonates by using CPA. In order to convert this method to a more simple and inexpensive test, we used a polystyrene surface instead of ECM-coated CPA plates [20]. Such studies for the evaluation of platelet function under flow conditions have not yet been performed with cord blood, either for full-term or for preterm infants.

Materials and Methods

Patients

All preterm infants (≤35 weeks' gestation) or full-term newborns (≥37 weeks' gestation) born at the Sheba Medical Center, Israel, between March 2003 and January 2004 were eligible for the study, provided their parents agreed to cord blood sampling. The blood samples were taken from the umbilical cord immediately after clamping using plastic syringes and quickly transferred to plastic tubes containing 1/10 vol trisodium citrate.

The medical history was obtained. Details were recorded from maternal and infant medical charts. Maternal data included parity and gravida, maternal diseases and medications, any complications during pregnancy and delivery mode. Infant data included gestational age, birth weight, gender and Apgar score. Infants were followed until discharge and studied for any postnatal complications.

Procedure for the CPA

The CPA procedure involves placing 200-μl samples of citrated whole blood in polystyrene four-well plates (Nunc; Roskilde, Denmark). Blood is subjected to shear stress (1,800 1/s) for 2 min using a rotating Teflon cone, as described in detail previously [12]. The plates are washed with phosphate-buffered saline, stained with May-Grünwald and analyzed using an image analysis system (Galai, Migdal Haemek, Israel). Two quantifiable parameters of platelet function were evaluated: platelet adhesion, defined as the percentage of total area covered by platelets (surface coverage or SC), and platelet aggregation, defined as the average size (AS) of the bound objects (either aggregates or single platelets). The normal adult values in our laboratory are SC: 8–13% and AS: 28–34 μm^2.

Statistical Analysis

Statistical analyses were carried out using the Statistical Program for Social Sciences (SPSS) Version 11.5 software. Patients' data were analyzed and compared to control group data using t tests, χ^2 test and analysis of variance and covariance with repeated measures, as required. Possible correlations between newborns' CPA (SC or AS) and various perinatal conditions and postnatal complications were evaluated using logistic regression. A p value of <0.05 was considered to be significant.

Ethics

The study was approved by the local ethics committee of our hospital in concordance with the Declaration of Helsinki. Informed parental consent was obtained for each participant.

Results

The study population comprised 29 preterm infants (≤35 weeks' gestation), and 160 full-term newborns (≥37 weeks' gestation) born at the Sheba Medical Center, Israel, during the study period.

The mean gestational ages of the preterm and full-term infants were 33.4 ± 1.1 and 39.0 ± 1.3 weeks, respectively, and their mean birth weights were 1,863.8 ± 286 and 3,328 ± 488 g, respectively. Platelet adhesion (SC) was lower in the preterm as compared to the full-term population (7.9 ± 3.6 vs. 9.2 ± 3.7%), with borderline statistical significance (p = 0.085). When linear regression was applied, significant correlation was found between SC and gestational age in all infants, as shown in figure 1 ($R^2 = 0.034$, p = 0.047).

Aggregation was similar in the preterm and full-term infants (mean AS: 24.2 ± 6.4 μm^2 in both groups). This value, however, is significantly lower than the normal adult values in our laboratory, which are AS: 28–34 μm^2.

No correlations were found between platelet function and gender or Apgar score of neonates. With respect to mode of delivery, similar SC was found among infants delivered by spontaneous vaginal delivery (n = 77 infants, SC: 8.9 ± 3.2%), cesarean section (n = 98, SC: 9.1 ± 4%) or instrumental delivery (vacuum/forceps, n = 14, SC: 9 ± 4.2%); however, AS was significantly higher in children born following assisted instrumental delivery as com-

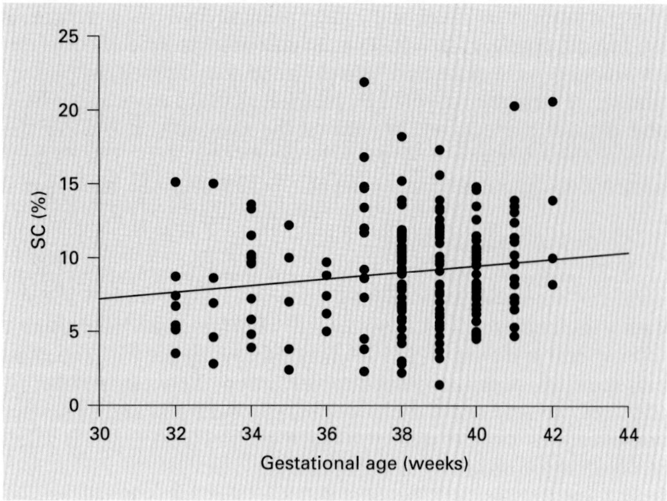

Fig. 1. SC as a function of gestational age.

Table 1. Impact of maternal prenatal conditions upon infantile CPA

	SC %	AS μm^2
PIH		
Yes (n = 4)	4.4 (1.7)*	22.8 (4.1)
No (n = 25)	8.4 (3.6)*	24.4 (6.7)
PMC		
Yes (n = 15)	8.5 (2.8)	25.4 (7.2)
No (n = 14)	7.2 (4.3)	22.9 (5.3)
PROM		
Yes (n = 4)	10.1 (4.0)	29.1 (7.2)
No (n = 25)	7.6 (3.5)	23.4 (6.0)

All values represent the mean with the SD in parentheses. * $p < 0.05$. PMC = Premature contractions; PROM = premature rapture of membranes.

pared to noncomplicated vaginal delivery (AS: 25.1 ± 6.2 compared to 23.2 ± 4.7 μm^2, p = 0.022).

Within the preterm group, platelet function was compared among infants with various prenatal maternal conditions, such as pregnancy-induced hypertension (PIH), premature contractions and premature rupture of membranes. We found lower SC in infants whose mothers suffered from PIH (p = 0.038; table 1). Logistic regression analysis confirmed the significance of maternal PIH as a factor affecting infant SC.

Among the full-term infants, 40 out of 160 neonates were born to mothers who reported the presence of some disease. Maternal diseases comprised a heterogeneous group, including gestational diabetes, hypothyroidism, premature contractions, asthma and urinary tract infection. No correlation was found between maternal disease and infantile CPA parameters within this group.

During follow-up we looked for the occurrence either of bleeding tendency or of postnatal complications, such as hyaline membrane disease (HMD), intraventricular hemorrhage (IVH), necrotizing enterocolitis or sepsis. None of the infants within our study group suffered any bleeding diathesis. Only one infant suffered from necrotizing enterocolitis, and one other infant suffered from sepsis. The CPA parameters of these 2 infants correlated with gestational age, and no further statistical analyses were performed for those single cases. Table 2 presents CPA results for infants with HMD (n = 6) and IVH (n = 3). Although lower SC was measured for infants who suffered IVH, the difference was not statistically significant when compared to healthy premature infants.

Table 2. Impact of HMD or IVH in premature infants upon CPA

	SC %	AS μm^2
HMD		
Yes (n = 6)	7.7 (3.4)	25.0 (9.0)
No (n = 23)	8.0 (3.8)	24.0 (5.7)
IVH		
Yes (n = 3)	6.7 (1.9)	28.8 (8.1)
No (n = 26)	8.1 (3.8)	23.7 (6.1)

All values represent mean with SD in parentheses. p value is nonsignificant.

Discussion

In our study, we demonstrated a significant correlation between SC, manifesting platelet adhesion, and gestational age in all infants. Previous studies of neonatal platelet function have demonstrated decreased response to most physiological agonists, including thrombin, combination of ADP and epinephrine and thromboxane A_2 (TxA_2) [8]. This hyporesponsiveness is believed to stem from transient physiological alterations of the neonatal hemostatic system. Some of these alterations recently studied include impaired platelet-dense granule release in neonates [7], a decreased number of GPIIb/IIIa receptors upon resting neonatal platelets, a defect of GPIb internalization [11, 21, 22], a reduced number of α-adrenergic receptors in newborn platelets [23] and deficient TxA_2 synthesis and response [24]. The poor response of neonatal platelets to TxA_2 may be related to impaired postreceptor signal transduction pathway [25, 26]. Interestingly, when compared to full-term neonatal platelets, the platelets obtained from premature neonates showed an even poorer response [9].

Studies of neonatal platelet function have been hampered by the need for relatively large volumes of blood in order to perform standardized studies. CPA is an attractive mode for rapid, feasible evaluation of platelet function in neonates using very small amounts of blood. The method has already been used for diagnostic purposes of various platelet disorders, including infant studies [12–19]. Whereas in previous studies, platelet adhesion and aggregation were examined on ECM, we used polystyrene surface instead of ECM-coated plates in order to make the method simpler and less expensive [20].

As indicated by our study, SC values measured by CPA correlated with gestational age and were lower for premature neonates as compared to term babies. A similar correlation was found in a previous study [18]. In our study, however, the values of SC measured are significantly lower compared to previous reference values (mean SC of full-term neonate 9.2 vs. 35.7% previously, mean SC of preterm infant 7.9 vs. 28.7% previously). The difference clearly stems from the use of polystyrene plates, which alters the method applied to test platelet adhesion.

Shenkman et al. [20] investigated platelet deposition on polystyrene surface compared with that on ECM under defined shear rates. Despite the higher shear rate applied, platelet deposition on polystyrene was less extensive than on ECM, with lower results of both SC and AS. However, a correlation between polystyrene and ECM was found for both AS and SC. The authors concluded that platelet adhesion to polystyrene is absolutely dependent on platelet activation, whereas even passive platelets with a low number of active receptors can adhere to ECM under high shear conditions. Therefore, it is possible that the enhanced ECM adhesion of neonatal platelets as compared to adult platelets is artificial. The increased neonatal platelet deposition on ECM surface under flow conditions has been explained by the role of the von Willebrand plasma factor [17]. The von Willebrand plasma factor is known to be more multimerized, and therefore more active in neonates than in adults [27, 28]. In our study, the SC of full-term infants was within the normal adult reference range for our laboratory (SC 8–13%) and slightly lower for preterm infants, as explained in concordance with previous studies [9].

With regard to platelet aggregation, the AS values of full-term neonates, preterm neonates and adults were similar while using the ECM surface. However, in the present study, the AS of neonates was lower than the normal adult values in our laboratory (mean neonatal AS 24.2 μm^2, while normal adult values are 28–34 μm^2). Platelet aggregation depends mainly on the GPIIb-IIIa receptor, which presents at lower levels in neonatal platelets compared to adults. This is compatible with previous studies that showed relative neonatal platelet function impairment [8, 9, 11, 23–26].

No correlations were found between platelet function and gender or between platelet function and Apgar score. With regard to mode of delivery, similar SC was found among infants delivered by spontaneous vaginal delivery, cesarean section or instrumental delivery (vacuum/forceps); however, AS was significantly higher in children born following assisted instrumental delivery as compared to noncomplicated vaginal delivery ($p = 0.022$; table 2). This finding may stem from hyperstimulation of neonatal platelets during such labor or from perinatal stress reaction.

Maternal conditions did not affect infantile CPA, apart from infants born to mothers with PIH, whose SC was significantly lower. This finding deserves further attention and should be ascertained by further population studies.

Correlations with postnatal complications were also investigated. Sick infants may present with hemostatic alterations, including activation of the coagulation and fibrinolytic systems accompanied by consumptive coagulopathy [29]. Previous studies indicate that platelet adhesion as measured by SC is poorer in either septic preterm infants or preterm infants with HMD than in healthy preterm infants [18, 19]. Naturally, we assumed that initially detected poorer platelet function may be associated with higher infant morbidity. Nevertheless, in the present study, there were only 6 preterm infants with HMD and 3 with IVH. No statistically significant difference was noted in these infants as compared to healthy premature infants. Intracranial hemorrhage may be the presenting symptom of some severe coagulation deficiencies [30–32]. On the other hand, it has recently been suggested that IVH may be associated with infantile thrombophilia, triggering vessel occlusion and high pressure bleeding. The association of IVH and presence of factor V Leiden was reported in two case series [33, 34]; however, a previous prospective study by our group did not support this finding [35]. Among infants with IVH in the present study group lower SC values were measured, yet statistical significance was not detected; thus the predictive value of CPA could not be elucidated. This is probably due to the small number of sick preterm infants, also stemming from the fact that the mean gestational age of the preterm infants was 33.4 weeks (± 1.1). Technical difficulties were encountered in sampling cord blood of younger preterm neonates. Further studies are required in order to elucidate the possible correlation between CPA-tested neonatal platelet function and perinatal and postnatal complications.

References

1 Nathan D, Orkin S: Nathan and Oski's Hematology of Infancy and Childhood, ed 6. Philadelphia, WB Saunders, 2003.
2 Andrew M, Paes B, Milner M: Development of human coagulation system in the full term infant. Blood 1987;70:165–172.
3 Andrew M, Paes B, Milner M: Development of human coagulation system in healthy premature infant. Blood 1988;72:1651–1657.
4 Aballi AJ, de Lamerens S: Coagulation changes in the neonatal period and in early infancy. Pediatr Clin North Am 1962;9:785–817.
5 Andrew M, Kelton J: Neonatal thrombocytopenia. Clin Perinatol 1984;11:359–391.
6 Arad ID, Alpan G, Sznajderrman SD, Eldor A: The mean platelet volume in the neonatal period. Am J Perinatol 1986;3:1–3.
7 Mankin P, Marngos J, Akhand M, Saving KL: Impaired platelet dense granules release in neonate. J Pediatr Hematol Oncol 2000;22:143–147.
8 Rajasekhar D, Kestin A, Bednarek F: Neonatal platelets are less reactive than adult platelets to physiological agonists in whole blood. Thromb Haemost 1994;72:957–963.
9 Rajasekhar D, Barnard M, Francis J, Bednarek F: Platelet hyporeactivity in very low birth weight neonates. Thromb Haemost 1997;77:1002–1007.
10 Simak J, Holada K, Janota J, Stranak Z: Surface expression of major membrane glycoproteins on resting and TRAP-activated neonatal platelets. Pediatr Res 1999;46 445–449.
11 Hezard N, Potron G, Schlegel N, Amory C, Leroux B, Nguyen P: Unexpected persistence of platelet hyporeactivity beyond the neonatal period: a flow cytometric study in neonates, infants and older children. Thromb Haemost 2003;90:116–123.
12 Varon D, Dardik R, Shenkman B, Kotev-Emeth S, Farzame N, Tamarin I, Savion N: A new method for quantitative analysis of whole blood platelet interaction with extracellular matrix under flow conditions. Thromb Res 1997;85:283–294.
13 Knobler H, Savion N, Shenkman B, Kotev-Emeth S, Varon D: Shear induced platelet adhesion and aggregation on subendothelium are increased in diabetic patients. Thromb Res 1998;90:181–190.
14 Kennet G, Lubetsky A, Shenkman B, Tamarin I, Dardik R, Rechavi A, Barzilai A, Martinowitz U, Savion N, Varon D: Cone and platelet analyzer (CPA): a new test for prediction of bleeding among thrombocytopenic patients. Br J Haematol 1998;101:255–259.
15 Shenkman B, Rubinstein E, Tamarin I, Dardik R, Savion N, Varon D: Activated platelets mediate *Staphylococcus aureus* deposition on subendothelial extracellular matrix: the role of glycoprotein Ib. Platelets 1999;10:36–44.
16 Dardik R, Kaufmann Y, Savion N, Rosenberg N, Shenkman B, Varon D: Platelets mediate tumor cell adhesion to the subendothelium under flow conditions: involvement of platelet GPIIbIIIa and tumor cell integrins. Int J Cancer 1997;70:201–207.
17 Shenkman B, Linder N, Savion N, Dardik R, Kennet G, German B, Varon D: Increased neonatal platelet deposition on subendothelium under flow conditions: the role of plasma von Willebrand factor. Pediatr Res 1999;45:270–275.
18 Linder N, Shenkman B, Levin E, Sirota L, Tamarin I, Dardik R, Lubin D, Savion N, Varon D: Deposition of whole blood platelet on extracellular matrix under flow conditions in preterm infants. Arch Dis Child 2002;86:127–130.
19 Finkelstein Y, Shenkman B, Sirota L, Vishne TH, Dardik R, Varon D, Linder N: Whole blood platelet deposition on extracellular matrix under flow conditions in preterm neonatal sepsis. Eur J Pediatr 2002;161:270–274.
20 Shenkman B, Savion N, Tamarin I, Dardik R, Varon D: Testing of platelet deposition on polystyrene surface under flow conditions by cone and platelet analyzer: the role of platelet activation, fibrinogen and von Willebrand factor. Thromb Res 2000;99:353–361.
21 Kuhne T, Ryan G, Blanchette V, Kuhne T, Ryan G, Blanchette V, Semple JW, Hornstein A, Mody M, Chang W, McWhirter L, Freedman J: Platelet surface glycoproteins in healthy and preeclamptic mothers and their newborn infants. Pediatr Res 1996;40:876–880.
22 Sitaru AG, Holzhauer S, Speer GP, Singer D, Obergfell A, Waller U, Grossman R: Neonatal platelets from cord blood and peripheral blood. Platelets 2005;16:203–210.
23 Corby DG, O'Barr TP: Decreased alpha-adrenergic receptors in newborn platelets: cause of abnormal response to epinephrine. Dev Pharmacol Ther 1981;2:215–225.
24 Israels SJ, Odaibo FS, Robertson C, McMillan EM, McNicol A: Deficient thromboxane synthesis and response in platelets from premature infants. Pediatr Res 1997;41:218–223.
25 Israels SJ, Cheang T, Robertson C, McMillan-Ward EM, McNicol A: Impaired signal transduction in neonatal platelets. Pediatr Res 1999;45:687–691.
26 Gelman B, Setty BNY, Chen D, Amin-Hanjani S, Stuart MJ: Impaired mobilization of intracellular calcium in neonatal platelets. Pediatr Res 1996;39:692–696.
27 Katz JA, Moake JL, McPherson PD, Weinstein MJ, Moise KJ, Carpenter RJ, Sala DJ: Relationship between human development and disappearance of unusually large von Willebrand factor multimers from plasma. Blood 1989;73:1851–1858.
28 Weinstein MJ, Blanchard R, Moake JL, Vosburgh E, Moise K: Fetal and neonatal von Willebrand factor (VWF) is unusually large and similar to the VWF in patients with thrombotic thrombocytopenic purpura. Br J Haematol 1989;72:68–72.
29 Aronis S, Platokouki H, Photopoulos S, Adamtziki E, Xanthou M: Indications of coagulation and/or fibrinolytic system activation in healthy and sick very low birth weight infants. Biol Neonate 1998;74:337–344.
30 Yoffe G, Buchanan GR: Intracranial hemorrhage in newborn and young infants with hemophilia. J Pediatr 1988;113:333.
31 Abbondanzo SL, Gootenberg JE, Lofts R, McPherson R: Intracranial hemorrhage in congenital deficiency of FXIII. Am J Pediatr Hematol Oncol 1988;10:65–68.
32 Struwe FE: Intracranial hemorrhage and occlusive hydrocephalus in hereditary bleeding disorders. Dev Med Child Neurol 1970;12:165.
33 Pet J, Hiltunen L, Felman V: Increased risk of intraventricular hemorrhage in preterm infants with thrombophilia. Pediatr Res 2001;49:643–646.
34 Riikonen R, Kekomaki R: Resistance to activated protein C in childhood hydrocephalus. Thromb Haemost 1998;79:1059–1060.
35 Kenet G, Maayan-Metzger A, Rosenberg N, Sela BA, Mazkereth R, Ifrah A, Kuint J: Thrombophilia does not increase risk for neonatal complications in preterm infants. Thromb Haemost 2003;90:823–828.

Acta Haematologica

Acta Haematol 2006;115:157–161
DOI: 10.1159/000090929

Maternal Selective Serotonin Reuptake Inhibitor Intake Does Not Seem to Affect Neonatal Platelet Function Tests

A. Maayan-Metzger[a] J. Kuint[a] A. Lubetsky[b] B. Shenkman[b] R. Mazkereth[a] G. Kenet[b]

[a]Department of Neonatology, The Edmond and Lily Safra Children's Hospital and [b]Pediatric Coagulation Service, National Hemophilia Center and Institute of Thrombosis and Hemostasis, Sheba Medical Center, Tel Hashomer and Sackler Faculty of Medicine, Tel Aviv University, Tel Hashomer, Israel

Key Words

Platelet function · Selective serotonin reuptake inhibitors

Abstract

Recently, concerns have been raised regarding the potential impairment of neonatal platelet function and the potential risk of bleeding in neonates born to mothers treated with selective serotonin reuptake inhibitors (SSRI). Our aim was to test whether the platelet function of neonates born to SSRI-treated mothers was impaired when compared to non-SSRI-exposed neonates. In a single-center prospective study, platelet function was evaluated using a cone and platelet analyzer (CPA) device and compared between mother-infant pairs as well as normal non-SSRI-exposed infants. Twenty-seven SSRI-exposed and 27 non-SSRI-exposed full-term neonates and their 23 mothers were tested. No correlation was found between SSRI exposure among either neonates or mothers and parameters of surface coverage (SC) and average size (AS), manifesting platelet function as tested by CPA. SC was similar among SSRI-exposed babies as compared to those in the control group, whereas the size of platelet aggregates (AS) was higher among controls. Neither maternal diseases nor SSRI intake were associated with impaired platelet function and lower SC values, nor were any perinatal conditions. None of the babies suffered from bleeding. We conclude that maternal SSRI therapy does not impair whole-blood CPA-tested platelet function of healthy full-term neonates.

Introduction

Selective serotonin reuptake inhibitors (SSRIs) are currently administered as a first-line treatment for depression, as they have a favorable side effect profile. SSRI therapy is commonly used among pregnant women. Indeed, evidence has shown that there is no increased risk of congenital malformations in the newborns of SSRI-treated mothers, nor is there a tendency for premature labor [1–3]. Nevertheless, newborns of SSRI-treated mothers have presented with various clinical manifestations, such as irritability, jitteriness, increased muscle tone, respiratory distress, feeding difficulties, sleeping problems and convulsions [4, 5]. These manifestations indicate that the drug may cross the placenta and accumulate in the fetal blood, resulting in significant clinical postnatal symptoms. In contrast to this hypothesis, in a prospective series studying breast-fed babies born to

KARGER

Fax +41 61 306 12 34
E-Mail karger@karger.ch
www.karger.com

0001–5792/06/1154–0157$23.50/0

Accessible online at:
www.karger.com/aha

Ayala Maayan-Metzger, MD
Department of Neonatology
Sheba Medical Center
Tel Hashomer, 52621 (Israel)
Tel. +972 3 530 2424, Fax +972 3 530 2215, E-Mail maayan@post.tau.ac.il

mothers treated with SSRIs, low drug levels were recorded, as was an absence of abnormal clinical manifestations [6]. Due to the paucity of information available, the issue of potential toxicity and complications in newborns after maternal treatment with SSRI during the third trimester of pregnancy remains to be solved.

Recently, concerns have been raised regarding the effect of SSRIs on platelet aggregation, and hence the risk for bleeding. In depressed adults treated with SSRIs, studies regarding platelet function were not conclusive. Some studies showed a marked decrease in platelet serotonin, inhibition of plug formation and disturbed platelet aggregation [7, 8]. Other studies failed to show impaired platelet aggregation or any bleeding tendency [9, 10]. Measurements of platelet aggregation and 5-HT [5-hydroxytryptamine (serotonin) transporter] levels in babies have been described in only a few studies [11–14]. In breast-fed babies of mothers treated with SSRIs, no significant differences were recorded in 5-HT levels before and during maternal SSRI treatment [15]. Nevertheless, another study described acute bleeding in children treated with SSRIs [16] and even severe intraventricular hemorrhage in a full-term newborn whose mother had been treated with SSRI during pregnancy [17].

To the best of our knowledge, no studies have been published regarding platelet aggregation in newborns of mothers treated with SSRIs during pregnancy. Cone platelet aggregation (CPA) has been shown to be a reliable test for measuring platelet adhesion and aggregation. The use of a small amount of whole blood under flow conditions enables diagnosis of platelet function disorders [14, 18], von Willebrand disease and other coagulation abnormalities [19], and is an extremely attractive method for evaluating primary hemostasis in neonates [20].

The purpose of the current study is to estimate platelet function among full-term newborns born to mothers treated with SSRIs during pregnancy using the CPA measurement and to compare this measure with maternal platelet function and with healthy newborn controls.

Methods

During a period of 1 year (May 1, 2003, to May 31, 2004), 10,356 babies were born at the Sheba Medical Center. In this period, 49 mothers reported SSRI treatment during the last month of pregnancy.

According to the routine procedure, every newborn of a mother treated with SSRI at the end of her pregnancy is hospitalized in the newborn nursery for monitoring and observation for 4 days after birth.

Patients

The study group included 27 full-term newborns to mothers treated with one of the SSRI drugs during at least the last month of their pregnancy. These newborns were hospitalized for observation in the neonatology special care unit, and in order to study their platelet function, venous blood was drawn for CPA measurement during the first days of life, following parental consent. Clinical manifestations of bleeding were recorded. The control group consisted of 27 healthy full-term newborns matched to the study group in gestational age (GA). Cord blood for CPA was drawn immediately after birth. Due to the high volume of blood required for classical platelet aggregometry testing, neonatal platelet function in the study group and control infants was measured by the use of CPA only.

Details were recorded from the maternal anamnesis, infant medical charts and staff reports. Data included parity and gravida, maternal diseases, bleeding during pregnancy (nasal bleeding, gum bleeding and hematomas), delivery mode, type of SSRI taken (fluoxetine, paroxetine, citalopram hydrobromide), dose and time of last drug taken before delivery. Infant data included GA, birth weight, gender, Apgar score at 5 min, presence of meconium in amniotic fluid, and hematocrit level as taken routinely on the third day of life.

A venous blood sample for CPA and platelet functions was drawn from the mothers of the babies in the study group who agreed to the procedure (23 mothers) within 1–3 days following labor.

Laboratory Tests: CPA and Platelet Function Measurements

Blood was obtained by venipuncture of the mother's antecubital vein, using siliconized vacutainer tubes containing 1/10 vol citrate. Neonatal control blood samples were collected from cord blood immediately after clamping, whereas neonatal blood from infants of SSRI-treated mothers was obtained by venipuncture at days 1–3 following birth. Maternal platelet function tests were performed using standard aggregometry techniques to evaluate aggregation of platelet-rich plasma in the presence of known platelet agonists: ADP, collagen, epinephrine and ristocetin [12]. The percent (%T) at maximal aggregation was measured for each of these agonists. Within 3 min of collection, 250-μl aliquots of blood were added to polystyrene four-well plates (Nunc; Roskilde, Denmark) and then subjected to shear stress in the CPA [14] for 2 min. The plates were stained, washed and analyzed, as previously described [14], to yield quantifiable parameters of surface coverage (SC, %) and average size (AS, μm^2), correlating with platelet adhesion and aggregation. The recently checked normal values for full-term neonates (n = 160) are compatible with previously published adult values of SC (9.2 ± 3.7%) as well as AS (24.2 ± 5.8 μm^2), respectively [21]. The normal adult values are SC: 8–13% and AS: 28–34 μm^2 [14, 18–20].

Statistical Analysis

Statistical analysis was performed using the Statistical Program for Social Sciences (SPSS) version 11.0 software (Chicago, Ill., USA). Patient data were analyzed and compared to data from our control group using χ^2 test and t tests (for continuous data). Possible associations between the baby's CPA (SC or AS) and various perinatal conditions and parameters were evaluated by logistic regression, using a cutoff point of 5.5% [1 standard deviation below the mean SC for neonates; see 21] for SC to differentiate between normal or low CPA infants. The conditions and parameters evaluated included the following: GA, birth weight, gender, Apgar score, maternal diseases, meconium-stained amniotic fluid, maternal bleeding diathesis during pregnancy, delivery mode, infant's age at blood CPA sampling, time of maternal drug withdrawal before delivery, and SSRI type or dose. A two-sided two-tailed p value of <0.05 was considered significant.

Results

Table 1 presents the data from the study and control groups. The two groups were similar with regard to GA, delivery mode, birth weight, gender, Apgar score at 5 min, and hematocrit. Among both groups, maternal diseases were similar and included gestational diabetes, hypothyroidism, premature contractions and urinary tract infection.

The average CPA-SC was similar in the study and control groups. Indeed, the CPA-AS score was even higher in the study than in the control group (table 1), but was within the normal values in both groups. In 2 babies from the study group and 4 in the control group, the CPA-SC score was lower than 6%, a level considered low in healthy adults [14, 18–20] as well as in neonates (see laboratory methods). In those 2 babies in the study group, therapy consisted of a nonsimilar type of SSRI drug. The SSRI dose was low (20 mg/day for each mother), and the time from drug withdrawal was 8 and 72 h before delivery, respectively. In both cases, the timing of blood sampling for CPA was within the first day of life.

Upon logistic regression, no association was found between infants with low CPA (SC or AS) and GA, birth weight, gender, Apgar score, maternal diseases, meconium-stained amniotic fluid, maternal bleeding, diathesis during pregnancy, delivery mode, infant's age at blood CPA sampling, time of maternal drug withdrawal before delivery, SSRI type or dose. In addition, no correlation was found between maternal and infant CPA.

None of the babies in the study group presented with clinical signs of active bleeding during the 4 days of intrahospital follow-up.

The mean maternal CPA-SC was 8.9 ± 0.7%. In 2 mothers, the levels were less than 6%. In these 2, the babies' CPA was higher than 6%, though the SSRI type was not similar. The SSRI dose in the women whose CPA-SC was the lowest (2.1%) was among the highest administered, i.e. 60 mg/day. In this case, maternal platelet functions were also disturbed. Standard platelet aggregation tests performed with several agonists (ADP, collagen, epinephrine and ristocetin) disclosed decreased aggregation in response to epinephrine, whereas the response with other agonists was normal. Serotonin release tests and measurements of 5-HT were not performed in our study.

Table 1. Data of the study and control groups

	Study group (n = 27)	Control group (n = 27)	p value
Gestational age[a], weeks	38.8 ± 1.17	38.8 ± 1.15	0.82
Birth weight[a], g	3,182 ± 472	3,236 ± 420	0.66
Male gender	14 (52)	17 (63)	0.27
Maternal parity[a]	1.74 ± 0.9	1.55 ± 1.62	0.61
Spontaneous delivery	18 (67)	18 (67)	0.23
Maternal diseases	3 (11)	5 (18.5)	0.58
Apgar at 5 min[a]	9.85 ± 0.36	9.96 ± 0.2	0.17
Hematocrit[a], %	54.3 ± 7.1	55.4 ± 6.3	0.55
CPA-SC, %			
Mean ± SD	10.44 ± 2.7	9.34 ± 3.3	0.19
Range	4.7 – 15.8	4.7 – 14.6	
CPA-AS, μm²			
Mean ± SD	27.9 ± 9	23.9 ± 6	0.056
Range	18.3 – 57	16.4 – 36.4	

Figures in parentheses represent percentage.
[a] Values represent mean ± SD.

No correlation was found between maternal CPA and hematocrit levels, maternal diseases, time of drug withdrawal, SSRI type and bleeding diathesis during pregnancy or labor. Higher SSRI doses correlated with lower CPA of the mothers tested but not with the CPA of their babies.

In 6 mothers, platelet function standard aggregation tests with epinephrine yielded lower than 30% response at maximal aggregation. In those mothers, the mean CPA-AS was lower than in those with normal platelet aggregometry (20.9 vs. 28.1 μm², respectively; p = 0.05). No correlations were found between disturbed platelet aggregometry tests and all other parameters measured.

Discussion

This study focused on the potential impairment of newborn platelet function following intrauterine exposure to SSRI.

The known prevalence of SSRI intake by pregnant women is about 0.5% of mothers and newborns in our institution. This may be an underestimation, since it must be assumed that not all women report SSRI use, so that the exact rate of SSRI use during pregnancy cannot be determined. In addition, increased legitimization of the use of antidepressant medication has already shown its impact though the increased use of such drugs among the general population, and may be expected to increase even further.

No correlation was found between maternal SSRI use and the infant's abnormal platelet function as measured by CPA. In accordance with previous studies that checked 5-HT levels in neonatal cord blood [22–25], we assumed the presence of SSRI in the blood of infants of mothers treated with SSRI; however, the levels of SSRI in neonatal blood were not directly evaluated in our study. Low CPA values were found among healthy newborn infants that were not exposed to SSRI during pregnancy.

Anderson et al. [22] found low 5-HT levels in the cord blood of full-term newborns without intrauterine exposure to SSRI. Levels of 5-HT in the newborns reached adult levels at the age of 1 month. The same study [22] showed low 5-HT levels in the cord blood of newborns of mothers treated with SSRI, as compared with babies whose mothers were not treated with SSRI. In our study, as already mentioned, no correlation was shown between maternal SSRI intake and neonatal SC; nevertheless, the CPA impairment noted in some healthy nonexposed babies could possibly be attributed to physiological neonatal platelet defects, such as lower 5-HT levels [22] that may affect platelet function.

Previous studies dealing with neonates born to mothers following SSRI intake showed that the presence of the drug in the newborn blood is unquestionable. Several studies reported various clinical presentations that were attributed to SSRI in the baby's blood as well as SSRI withdrawal symptoms [4, 5, 26]. Laine et al. [23] found a 4-fold increase in serotonergic symptom score, in particular tremors, irritability and rigidity, among newborns to SSRI-treated mothers compared with controls. Nevertheless, evidence of the drug's impact upon the baby's coagulation has not yet been established. Coagulation measurement is not routinely performed at most centers, and its necessity should be determined. Reports of bleeding in the neonatal period among these newborns are extremely rare [17], which correlates with our finding that primary hemostasis as tested by CPA was not affected in our study group. Those babies born to SSRI-treated mothers were not at risk compared to healthy controls, and neither platelet function test impairment nor clinical bleeding symptoms were noted.

In our study group, venous blood was withdrawn for CPA tests within 1–3 days of age. Results were compared with cord blood taken from the controls and analyzed for CPA. Despite the difference in blood sampling methods, it can be assumed that CPA results are comparable, since the life span of platelets is longer than 3 days, and the half-life of SSRIs is sufficiently long (2.9–7 days) to maintain its potential impact upon neonatal platelets within the first days of life [24]. This assumption is supported by the study of Laine et al. [23], which revealed similar or only slightly (not significantly) lower drug concentrations on the second day of life as compared to umbilical cord drug concentrations in newborns of SSRI-treated mothers. Thus, if platelet functions were impaired, this would have been similarly reflected in cord blood and in venous blood as well, when tested within the first days of life.

Evaluation of platelet function in the neonatal period is troublesome and requires special attention. Standard platelet aggregation tests or studies of cord-blood-derived platelets using monoclonal antibodies and flow cytometry techniques generally report the hyporesponsiveness of neonatal platelets [10–13, 25]. The duration of platelet hyporeactivity and its clinical significance have not yet been completely elucidated [25]. The use of CPA to evaluate platelet function of neonates has previously been reported [20] in a study applying CPA either to neonatal cord blood samples or to neonatal venous blood. Neonatal platelet function test results were similar, regardless of blood sampling technique. The potential interpretation of platelet function using very small amounts of venous blood or cord blood makes CPA testing an attractive method for rapid, feasible evaluation of platelet function in neonates and a candidate test that may be applied to resolve issues such as the therapeutic impact of maternally obtained drugs upon neonatal platelets.

Maternal SSRI therapy may impair their platelet function [7, 8]; however, such impairment has not been evaluated using CPA measurements before. Since neonatal platelet function in our study was tested by CPA, maternal CPA tests were obtained as well along with classic aggregometry measured for SSRI-treated mothers. Although this study focused on the newborn babies and the impact of potential coagulation abnormalities due to maternal SSRI use, we found that 2 of the mothers had low recorded CPA and 6 had abnormal platelet aggregation with epinephrine. These findings, in a small subgroup of SSRI-treated mothers, deserve further attention to discover whether such a decrease in platelet function is a significant finding either in pregnancy and/or following labor, and whether these laboratory abnormalities may be associated with any potential predictive clinical coagulopathy.

In summary, we believe that CPA may serve as a potential test to rapidly and efficiently evaluate neonatal platelet function. Maternal SSRI intake was not associated with platelet function impairment (as tested by CPA) or with any bleeding symptoms in healthy full-term babies perinatally exposed to the drug in our study group. The potential impact of SSRI upon maternal platelet function and the predictive value of CPA with regard to delivery-associated bleeding complications of mothers, as well as the impact of SSRI exposure upon premature babies deserve consideration and require prospective data collection and further studies.

References

1 Kulin NA, Pastuszak A, Sage SR, Schick-Boschetto B, Spivey G, Feldkamp M, Ormond K, Matsui D, Stein-Schechman AK, Cook L, Brochu J, Rieder M, Koren G: Pregnancy outcome following maternal use of the new selective serotonin reuptake inhibitors: a prospective controlled multicenter study. JAMA 1998;279:609–610.
2 Hendrick V, Smith LM, Suri R, Hwang S, Haynes D, Altshuler L: Birth outcomes after prenatal exposure to antidepressant medication. Am J Obstet Gynecol 2003;188:812–815.
3 Goldstein DJ: Effects of third trimester fluoxetine exposure on the newborn. J Clin Psychopharmacol 1995;15:417–420.
4 Costei AM, Kozer E, Ho T, Ito S, Koren G: Perinatal outcome following third trimester exposure to paroxetine. Arch Pediatr Adolesc Med 2002;156:1129–1132.
5 Nordeng H, Lindemann R, Perminov KV, Reikvam A: Neonatal withdrawal syndrome after in utero exposure to selective serotonin reuptake inhibitors. Acta Paediatr 2001;90:288–291.
6 Piontek CM, Wisner KL, Perel JM, Peindl KS: Serum fluvoxamine levels in breastfed infants. J Clin Psychiatry 2001;62:111–113.
7 Hergovich N, Aigner M, Eichler HG, Entlicher J, Drucker C, Jilma B: Paroxetine decreases platelet serotonin storage and platelet function in human beings. Clin Pharmacol Ther 2000;68:435–442.
8 Alderman CP, Moritz CK, Ben-Tovim DI: Abnormal platelet aggregation associated with fluoxetine therapy. Ann Pharmacother 1992;26:1517–1579.
9 Alderman CP, Seshadri P, Ben-Tovim DI: Effects of serotonin reuptake inhibitors on hemostasis. Ann Pharmacother 1996;30:1232–1234.
10 Layton D, Clark DW, Pearce GL, Shakir SA: Is there an association between selective serotonin reuptake inhibitors and risk of abnormal bleeding? Results from a cohort study based on prescription event monitoring in England. Eur J Clin Pharmacol 2001;57:167–176.
11 Mankin P, Marngos J, Akhand M, Saving KL: Impaired platelet dense granules release in neonate. J Pediatr Hematol Oncol 2000;22:143–147.
12 Rajasekhar D, Kestin A, Bednarek F: Neonatal platelets are less reactive than adult platelets to physiological agonists in whole blood. Thromb Haemost 1994;72:957–963.
13 Simak J, Holada K, Janota J, Stranak Z: Surface expression of major membrane glycoproteins on resting and TRAP-activated neonatal platelets. Pediatr Res 1999;46:445–449.
14 Varon D, Dardik R, Shenkman B, Kotev-Emeth S, Farzame N, Tamarin I, Savion N: A new method for quantitative analysis of whole blood platelet interaction with extracellular matrix under flow conditions. Thromb Res 1997;85:283–294.
15 Epperson CN, Jatlow PI, Czarkowski K, Anderson GM: Maternal fluoxetine treatment in the postpartum period: effects on platelet serotonin and plasma drug levels in breastfeeding mother-infant pairs. Pediatrics 2003;112:e425.
16 Lake MB, Birmaher B, Wassick S, Mathos K, Yelovich AK: Bleeding and selective serotonin reuptake inhibitors in childhood and adolescence. J Child Adolesc Psychopharmacol 2000;10:35–38.
17 Duijvestijn YC, Kalmeijer MD, Passier AL, Dahlem P, Smiers F: Neonatal intraventricular haemorrhage associated with maternal use of paroxetine. Br J Clin Pharmacol 2003;56:581–582.
18 Knobler H, Savion N, Shenkman B, Kotev-Emeth S, Varon D: Shear induced platelet adhesion and aggregation on subendothelium are increased in diabetic patients. Thromb Res 1998;90:181–190.
19 Kennet G, Lubetsky A, Shenkman B, Tamarin I, Dardik R, Rechavi A, Barzilai A, Martinowitz U, Savion N, Varon D: Cone and platelet analyzer (CPA): a new test for prediction of bleeding among thrombocytopenic patients. Br J Haematol 1998;101:255–259.
20 Shenkman B, Linder N, Savion N, Dardik R, Kennet G, German B, Varon D: Increased neonatal platelet deposition on subendothelium under flow conditions: the role of plasma von Willebrand factor. Pediatr Res 1999;45:270–275.
21 Levy-Shraga Y, Maayan-Metzger A, Lubetsky A, Shenkman B, Kuint J, Martinowitz U, Kenet G: Platelet function of newborns as tested by cone and plate(let) analyzer correlates with gestational age. Acta Haematol 2006;115:152–156.
22 Anderson GM, Czarkowski K, Ravski N, Epperson CN: Platelet serotonin in newborns and infants: ontogeny, heritability, and effect of in utero exposure to selective serotonin reuptake inhibitors. Pediatr Res 2004;56:418–422.
23 Laine K, Heikkinen T, Ekblad U, Kero P: Effects of exposure to selective serotonin reuptake inhibitors during pregnancy on serotonergic symptoms in newborns and cord blood monoamine and prolactin concentrations. Arch Gen Psychiatry 2003;60:720–726.
24 Liston HL, DeVane CL, Boulton DW, Risch SC, Markowitz JS, Goldman J: Differential time course of cytochrome P450 2D6 enzyme inhibition by fluoxetine, sertraline, and paroxetine in healthy volunteers. J Clin Pharmacol 2002;22:169–173.
25 Hezard N, Potron G, Schlegel N, Amory C, Leroux B, Nguyen P: Unexpected persistence of platelet hyporeactivity beyond the neonatal period: a flow cytometric study in neonates, infants and older children. Thromb Haemost 2003;90:116–123.
26 Zeskind PS, Stephens LE: Maternal selective serotonin reuptake inhibitor use during pregnancy and newborn neurobehavior. Pediatrics 2004;113:368–375.

Acta Hæmatologica

Acta Haematol 2006;115:162–171
DOI: 10.1159/000090930

Current Issues in Prophylactic Therapy for Persons with Hemophilia

Amy L. Dunn Thomas C. Abshire

AFLAC Cancer Center and Blood Disorders Service, Department of Pediatrics, Emory University and Children's Healthcare of Atlanta, Atlanta, Ga., USA

Key Words
Hemophilia · Prophylaxis · Arthropathy

Abstract
Factor VIII or IX replacement in a prophylactic manner is utilized for many patients with moderate to severe hemophilia A or B. Studies have shown it to be effective in reducing or preventing degenerative joint disease in many but not all patients. However, many unanswered questions still exist and optimization of this expensive treatment regimen is needed. This paper recounts the current products that are available for use and explores the literature regarding different treatment regimens. It explores age at initiation, dose, interval between infusions, joint health outcomes, barriers to compliance and age at discontinuation of prophylaxis. Individualized treatment is recommended. Collaborative efforts are needed to improve outcomes for all persons with hemophilia.

Introduction

Congenital hemophilia results from absence or deficiency of factor VIII (FVIII) in classical hemophilia A, or of factor IX (FIX) in hemophilia B also known as Christmas disease. Hemophilia A and B are both X-linked recessive disorders. Hemophilia A has an incidence of approximately 1:10,000 people and hemophilia B 1:60,000 people [1, 2]. This group of disorders has been clinically recognized for nearly 2,000 years, but it was only recently with the availability of purified clotting factor replacement therapy that effective treatment for bleeding episodes became available. The hallmark of hemophilia-related bleeding is intra-articular bleeding. Joint-related morbidity remains the largest source of disability for persons with hemophilia. When clotting factor became available, on-demand infusions to treat bleeding episodes became the mainstay of treatment for patients with hemophilia. The concept of utilizing factor infusions to prevent bleeding episodes was introduced in Sweden in 1958 [3]. Since that time, using factor replacement in this prophylactic manner is increasingly utilized in developed countries. This chapter will briefly explore the history of hemophilia and concentrate on the role of factor prophylaxis in the treatment of persons with hemophilia. Existing literature on issues such as factor dosing strategies will be explored. Additionally, when to initiate and discontinue prophylaxis will be discussed. Available lit-

KARGER

Fax +41 61 306 12 34
E-Mail karger@karger.ch
www.karger.com

0001–5792/06/1154–0162$23.50/0

Accessible online at:
www.karger.com/aha

Amy L. Dunn, MD
AFLAC Cancer Center and Blood Disorders Service, Emory University
2015 Uppergate Drive NE, 4th floor, Atlanta, GA 30322 (USA)
Tel. +1 404 785 0908, Fax +1 404 727 4455
E-Mail amy.dunn@choa.org or Tabshir@emory.edu

Table 1. Effectiveness of pathogen attenuation in factor products

Procedure	Viruses		Prions	Emerging pathogens
	lipid-enveloped	non-lipid-enveloped		
Solvent detergent	High	None	Unknown	Unknown
Immunoaffinity chromatography	High	High	Moderate	Unpredictable
Ion exchange chromatography	High	High	Moderate	Unpredictable
Nano-/ultrafiltration	High	Moderate	Somewhat	Unpredictable

erature regarding outcomes of patients on long-term prophylaxis particularly focusing on joint function will be reviewed. Barriers to prophylaxis such as lack of peripheral venous access, compliance, factor availability and cost will be considered.

History

The first recorded reference to hemophilia occurred in the *Talmud*, a collection of Jewish writings and laws in the 2nd century AD. A male infant's circumcision was delayed if two brothers died as a result of bleeding [4]. Dr. John Conrad Otto of Philadelphia in 1803 accurately described the sex-linked inheritance of 'a hemorrhagic disposition existing in certain families' [5]. The assumption that two forms of hemophilia existed was made in 1944 when plasma samples from two different persons with hemophilia were mixed and the clotting times normalized [6]. In 1952 Steven Christmas, a young Canadian boy, was the first to be diagnosed with what is now known to be hemophilia B [7]. An international committee then assigned the names hemophilia A to FVIII deficiency and hemophilia B to FIX deficiency.

The first whole blood transfusion to treat a patient with hemophilia occurred in 1840 [8]. In the 1960s a series of clotting proteins were recognized and the interactions between the various coagulation proteins in a 'cascade' or 'waterfall' were described and have recently been reviewed [9]. Recognition that decreased clotting proteins led to the bleeding tendency seen in persons with hemophilia led to replacement therapy options. Initially, patients received whole blood transfusions or plasma. Judith Graham Pool discovered the FVIII-rich fraction of blood known as cryoprecipitate in the 1960s leading to the first effective treatment of patients with classical hemophilia [10]. Later in the 1960s and 1970s lyophilized FVIII and FIX concentrates became available for home use. This allowed the hemophilia population easier access to home therapy and a greater degree of independence. Tragically in the 1980s and 1990s many persons became infected with hepatitis or HIV as a result of contaminated products. Subsequently, viral inactivation of HIV and then HCV in the mid to late 1980s led to safer plasma-derived products. Development of recombinant products and viral attenuation steps for plasma-derived products in the last decade led to improved patient confidence and greater viral safety. Newer reconstitution systems and smaller diluent volumes for some products have led to increased convenience.

Plasma Products

Fresh-frozen plasma (FFP) is obtained by separating whole blood from many donors into the cellular portion and the plasma portion that is rich in coagulation proteins. Small and inconsistent amounts of FVIII and FIX are present in FFP making it substandard for treatment of hemophilia. FFP that is frozen, then thawed at 1–6°C results in a cold-resistant precipitant that is rich in FVIII, known as cryoprecipitate. Plasma is now routinely fractionated into individual components (i.e. FVIII, FIX and albumin). These plasma-derived factor concentrates can undergo a series of viral attenuation steps. These steps and their potential effectiveness at eliminating pathogens are summarized in table 1. Solvent detergent processes inactivate lipid-enveloped viruses such as HIV, hepatitis B and hepatitis C. In addition to removing lipid-enveloped viruses, immunoaffinity and ion exchange chromatography processes remove non-lipid-enveloped viruses such as parvovirus and hepatitis A. Additionally, the process of lyophilization (freeze drying) removes additional hepatitis A. Current FVIII/IX plasma-derived products are now derived from monoclonal technology. Monoclonal antibody immunoaffinity is a chromatography procedure in which a column of beads coated with a monoclonal antibody is engineered to attach only FVIII or FIX

Table 2. Comparison of currently available recombinant factor products

Product		Host cell	Pathogen attenuation	Stabilizer	Reconstituted volume, ml
First-generation FVIII	Recombinate	CHO	IA IE	Human albumin	10
Second-generation FVIII	Helixate/Kogenate FS ReFacto	Baby hamster kidney (BHK) CHO	IA, IE, SD, UF IA, IE, SD, nanofiltration	Sucrose Sucrose	2.5 4
Third-generation FVIII	Advate	CHO	IA, IE, SD	Trehalose	5
FIX	BeneFIX	CHO	IA, UF	Sucrose Amino acids	5–10

IA = Immunoaffinity; IE = ion exchange; SD = solvent detergent; UF = ultrafiltration.

and remove unwanted proteins or infectious agents. These monoclonal products are then stabilized using human albumin.

Recombinant Products

The production process for all recombinant FVIII products now contains multiple steps to help ensure quality, purity, and viral safety. Table 2 compares the currently available recombinant products and their viral attenuation steps.

First-Generation Product

Initially, the human FVIII gene is inserted into a Chinese hamster ovary (CHO) cell. During the second fermentation step, the CHO cells are placed in an environment that stimulates their growth so a sufficient amount of FVIII can be harvested. During this step, human albumin, bovine albumin and insulin are added to help the growth process. While these proteins and nutrients are used in the fermentation process, they are not needed in the final product. The third step consists of purification procedures, a key one being a process known as monoclonal antibody immunoaffinity chromatography. The mixture from the fermentation process is poured down a glass column lined with a murine antibody that attracts the FVIII. As the FVIII attaches to this antibody column, the unnecessary ingredients and proteins flow through and are discarded. A solution is then washed down the column to separate the FVIII from the murine antibody so that purified FVIII remains. The fourth and final step is formulation. The purified FVIII molecule is unstable by itself, so a stabilizer is attached to retain activity and maintain shelf life. In the first-generation FVIII product, this stabilizer is human albumin. Although there have been no documented cases of viral- or prion-borne illness transmitted through human albumin, a theoretical risk exists that products containing any human or animal protein may transmit human or animal viruses. In an effort to reduce risk even further, pharmaceutical companies have made improvements in their manufacturing processes, resulting in what are known as second- and third-generation recombinant products. Baxter's product Recombinate is currently the only first-generation licensed product that is available. The volume of infusion is 10 ml/vial.

Second-Generation Products

With second-generation products, manufacturers try to eliminate or minimize the animal and human protein in the process and in the final product vial. In second-generation product production, human albumin but no other animal proteins are used as ingredients in the fermentation step. Instead, recombinant human insulin has replaced the bovine form, and no bovine albumin is used. The products are purified using solvent detergent, ion exchange chromatography and monoclonal antibody immunoaffinity chromatography and ultrafiltration. In the formulation process, no human albumin is added to stabilize the FVIII molecule. Instead via a licensed technique, sugars, salts, or amino acids are used as stabilizers. Theoretically, this reduction of animal or human protein minimizes the risk of transmission of infectious agents.

The available products are distributed as Kogenate FS (formulated with sucrose) and Helixate FS. The volume of infusion is 2.5 ml/vial.

In 2000 another second-generation product, ReFacto, lacking the B domain of the FVIII molecule, received FDA approval. The B domain is not necessary for coagulant activity and the resultant shorter molecule is secreted more efficiently from cell culture. This product is purified using solvent detergent, ion exchange chromatography, monoclonal antibody immunoaffinity chromatography and nanofiltration. ReFacto is best monitored in vivo utilizing a chromogenic assay or a ReFacto substrate as the standard in a one-stage clotting assay. One-stage assays not utilizing a B domain-deleted substrate will yield significantly lower (40–50%) results. The volume of infusion is 4 ml/vial. Additional modifications to this product have been undertaken, one of which is to remove human albumin completely from the manufacturing process. This new third-generation product is currently undergoing clinical trials.

Third-Generation Products

In 2003 the FDA licensed the first recombinant FVIII product, Advate (Baxter Pharmaceuticals), produced without the addition of human or animal proteins during cell culture, purification or final formulation. This product is purified using solvent detergent, ion exchange and immunoaffinity chromatography. Animal-derived monoclonal antibodies are integral to the immunoaffinity chromatography step, but not detectable in the final formulation. The volume of infusion is 5 ml/vial.

Recombinant Product Summary

Efficacy studies between all three generations of FVIII products are similar as are inhibitor development rates [11–14]. Third-generation products are theoretically safer as human and animal proteins are practically eliminated. There has not, however, been documented viral- or prion-based disease transmission from the first- or second-generation recombinant products.

Recombinant FIX

Recombinant FIX is produced from genetically engineered CHO cells in cell culture that contains no human or animal proteins. It undergoes purification via chromatography and membrane filtration and requires no human or animal protein for stabilization. The volume of infusion for low and mid-range dosing is 5 ml/vial and for high-range infusion it is 10 ml/vial.

Prophylaxis

Definition

Prophylaxis refers to regularly scheduled infusion of clotting factor concentrate. The goals of prophylaxis are several: to allow patients to maintain a more normal lifestyle, to prevent the majority of bleeding episodes, and to prevent joint disease. This concept was introduced in 1958 in Sweden [3]. The Medical and Scientific Advisory Committee to the National Hemophilia Foundation consider this to be the standard of care in developed countries [15]. The term primary prophylaxis refers to ongoing factor infusions from early childhood before the establishment of recurrent bleeding. Some institutions begin prophylaxis prior to the first joint bleed. Secondary prophylaxis typically refers to a defined period of infusions. This is commonly utilized around procedures or strenuous activities such as surgical intervention or camp. Longer-term secondary prophylaxis to combat the recurrent joint bleeding often seen in established joint disease is sometimes utilized.

Considerations

Many issues should be considered prior to instituting prophylactic therapy [16]. Among these are patient selection issues such as: Which patient/what severity of hemophilia should be targeted? What is the most appropriate time at which to begin prophylaxis? Should prophylaxis be instituted in all patients by a certain age or should one wait until a pattern of bleeding is established. How will the therapy be delivered, through peripheral veins or central venous access devices (CVADs)? What dose of factor is most appropriate? What dosing interval should be utilized? How do you judge the efficacy of prophylaxis via physical examination scales, radiographic imaging or bleeding frequency? Can prophylactic therapy be safely stopped at a certain age? How can barriers to compliance be reduced or eliminated? Many of these issues remain controversial. This review attempts to present the published literature addressing these areas.

Timing of Initiation

Two schools of thought exist on the issue of when to institute prophylaxis. The first is to begin prophylaxis during the second year of life if the patient is not bleeding

Table 3. Swedish experience with primary prophylaxis

	Present age, years				
	3–6	7–12	13–17	18–23	24–32
Patients, n	6	9	20	10	15
Start age, years	1.1	1.2	2.6	4.9	7
Joint bleeds/year	0.1	0.1	3	5.6	5
FVIII/FIX units × 10^3/kg/year	4.3	4–7.4	1.5–4.9	1.2–3.8	0.4–2.6
Orthopedic joint score	0	0	1.2	2.9	6.6
Radiologic joint score	0	0	4.8	14.2	20.6

All values are means.

or after the first joint bleed. Evidence shows that early introduction of prophylaxis can prevent arthropathy, but numbers in these studies are relatively small and treatment regimens vary (table 3) [17–20]. It is also important to realize that early introduction of prophylaxis may reduce the frequency of bleeding into other locations and reduce hospital visits [21]. A review of patients from the Dutch National Hemophilia Treatment Center suggests that radiographic scores worsen by 8% for each year that prophylaxis is postponed after the first joint bleed [20]. However, approximately 10–14% of patients with severe disease rarely manifest bleeding and may be overtreated by this approach [18, 22–24]. Additionally, earlier use of prophylaxis may increase lifetime cost of factor. Limited data suggest that early (<6 months of age) exposure to factor may increase the incidence of inhibitor development [24]. Another small study, however, does not suggest an increased risk of inhibitor formation [25].

The second standard approach to beginning prophylaxis is to wait until a pattern of bleeding is manifested. A small study has shown that institution of prophylaxis a bit later, around 3 years of age, can preserve joint structure [19]. The Dutch experience suggests that 50% of their patients could delay the initiation of prophylaxis by a minimum of 1.5 years if prophylaxis was started after the first joint bleed instead of starting at age 1 year [26]. Delaying initiation of therapy decreases cost and the likelihood of needing a CVAD [27]. One concern with this approach is that the amount of joint damage/inflammation initiated by even one or two bleeds may lead to slowly progressive arthropathy that takes years to recognize. All studies suggest that prophylactic therapy is superior to standard on-demand therapy in terms of joint outcomes [28–31]. An ongoing North American study is evaluating joint outcomes in patients started on early prophylaxis compared to a group who receives a more aggressive on-demand therapy, but results are not yet available. The Italians are pursuing a similar study comparing 3 times weekly prophylactic infusions of 25 U/kg to on-demand infusions of 25 U/kg given until resolution of each bleeding episode [32]. Preliminary results suggest that 13.8 bleeding events/person/year were avoided by prophylaxis compared to on-demand therapy.

Dosing

The Swedish and Dutch Hemophilia Treatment Centers have the longest follow-up of patients on different treatment doses of prophylaxis [33]. In Sweden patients are generally started around the age of 1 year of life on a high-dose regimen of 25–40 IU/kg 3 times a week for patients with FVIII deficiency and 2 times per week for those with FIX deficiency. In the Netherlands an intermediate-dose regimen is utilized, and patients with hemophilia A receive 15–25 IU/kg 2 or 3 times a week while those with hemophilia B receive 30–50 IU/kg 1 or 2 times per week [33]. In both centers dosages are adjusted based upon breakthrough bleeding. On average, patients treated via the high-dose regimen since 1980 were 3 years younger at the initiation of prophylaxis than those in the intermediate group. They were less likely to interrupt prophylaxis but were more likely to utilize a CVAD (12 vs. 3%). The age-adjusted use of factor concentrates was 2.19 times higher in the patient receiving high-dose infusions. On average 996 IU/kg/year was required to avoid one joint bleed. Patients receiving high-dose prophylaxis had fewer annual joint bleeds by 77% and lower radiographic scores by 33%. Treatment cost was significantly higher for patients on the high-dose therapy [34]. Length of follow-up was longer in the intermediate-dose group making these radiographic outcomes particularly difficult to compare directly. The difference in quality of life measures between the two groups did not achieve statistical significance.

Interval

The interval between dosing has been relatively noncontroversial until recently. Most regimens utilize an interval between infusions estimated or measured to keep the trough factor level activity ≥1%. As most patients with baseline levels ≥1% do not have severe arthropathy, this seemed a reasonable goal. Given standard half-life of 10–12 h for infused FVIII and 20–24 h for FIX this translates to two or three infusions weekly, respectively [35]. A recent study of recombinant FVIII suggests that in vivo recovery in children <6 years of age was lower (1.9 ± 0.4 compared to 2.4 ± 0.5 IU/dl/IU/kg) than in older patients (median age 18 years). In the same patient groups half-life was significantly shorter (9.7 ± 1.9 compared to 12 ± 4.3 h) in the younger age group [36]. Pharmacokinetic dosing based on individual patient response to therapy has been shown to reduce factor usage [37]. More recently preliminary data from Canada have suggested that higher dose factor given on a less frequent basis and then escalated based on bleeding patterns may be effective in reducing both bleeding rates and progressive arthropathy in some patients [38]. In the Canadian FVIII dose escalation study, patients are started on once a week infusions of 50 U/kg and the dosing is changed to twice a week infusions of 30 U/kg and then to every other day infusion of 25 U/kg if they suffered from recurrent bleeding. Thus far, only 36% of patients enrolled have proceeded to the twice a week infusions and only 16% to every other day [38].

Outcomes with Prophylaxis

Joint Bleeding Rates

Primary prophylaxis clearly reduces the rate of joint bleeding in most patients. Reduction in bleeding is tied not only to age at initiation of therapy but also to dose and interval as seen in table 1. In the largest study to date, joint bleeding rates were much lower: 5.65 as compared to 16.5 bleeds/year ($p < 0.00000$) in patients who received greater than 45 weeks/year of prophylaxis compared to patients on no specific prophylactic regimen [18]. Although long-term secondary prophylaxis also reduces the frequency of joint hemorrhages, retrospective results are not as dramatic as those seen with primary prophylaxis [17, 39–41]. One small prospective study of 13 boys showed that treatment with long-term secondary prophylaxis controlled recurrent joint bleeding in 12 of 13 boys [42]. One boy required surgical synovectomy due to recurrent bleeding and one proceeded to surgical synovec-

Table 4. World Federation of Haemophilia joint classification

Radiographic/Pettersson (0–13)		
Osteoporosis	Absent	0
	Present	1
Enlarged epiphysis	Absent	0
	Present	1
Irregular subchondral bone	Absent	0
	Partly involved	1
	Totally involved	2
Narrowing of joint space	Absent	0
	Joint space >1 mm	1
	Joint space <1 mm	2
Subchondral cyst formation	Absent	0
	1 cyst	1
	>1 cyst	2
Erosions at joint margins	Absent	0
	Present	1
Incongruence of joint surfaces	Absent	0
	Slight	1
	Pronounced	2
Joint deformity (angulation and/or displacement between the articulating bony ends)	Absent	0
	Slight	1
	Pronounced	2
Orthopedic score (0–20)		
Pain (0–3)		
0 No pain No functional deficit No analgesic use (except with hemarthrosis)		
1 Mild pain Does not interfere with occupation nor with ADL May require occasional nonnarcotic analgesic		
2 Moderate pain Partial or occasional interference with occupation or ADL May require occasional narcotics		
3 Severe pain Interferes with occupation or ADL Requires frequent use of nonnarcotic and narcotic medications		
Bleeding (0–3)		
0 None		
1 No major, 1–3 minor hemarthroses per year		
2 1–2 major or 4–6 minor hemarthroses per year		
3 3 or more major or 7 or more minor hemarthroses per year		
Clinical features (0–12)		
Swelling	Absent	0
	Present	2
Muscle atrophy	Absent	0
	Present	2
Axial deformity	Absent	0
	20–30° valgus (5° varus)	1
	>30° valgus (>5° varus)	2
Joint crepitus	Absent	0
	Present	1
ROM	<10% loss of total ROM	0
	10–30% loss	1
	>30% loss	2
Flexion contracture	≤15°	0
	>15°	2
Instability	Absent	0
	Present, function unaffected	1
	Present, interferes with function and may require bracing	2

ADL = Activities of daily living; ROM = range of movement.

tomy due to difficulty in adherence to scheduled infusions.

Radiographic Changes

Arnold and Hilgartner [43] have classified the radiographic presentation of degenerative changes, which occur in a stepwise fashion. Pettersson et al. [44] as seen in table 4 has offered an additional schema tabulating these worsening radiographic changes in conjunction with the clinical/orthopedic assessments adapted by the World Federation of Haemophilia (WFH) Orthopedic Advisory Committee. More recently magnetic resonance imaging (MRI) techniques have been utilized to evaluate hemophilic joint disease [45–47]. MRI seems to be most helpful in identifying clinically indeterminate joint disease and to assess the severity of synovitis prior to an intra-articular procedure [46]. An international effort is underway to standardize and validate a grading system utilizing MRI.

The Swedish have the longest and most extensive experience of the effect of primary prophylaxis on radiographically assessed joint disease, although only 15 patients were in the initial experience. In patients who began prophylaxis between 1 and 2 years of age and who received 25–40 U/kg of FVIII (3 times a week) or FIX (twice a week) no plain radiographic evidence (Pettersson) of joint disease was evident after long-term follow-up [17]. A German study that included 8 patients on primary prophylaxis had similar results [39]. In this study, patients who started prophylaxis at later ages had worse radiographic outcomes. The Dutch experience with infusions of a lower dose of 10–20 U/kg 3 times per week showed slightly higher joint scores than patients on a higher dose of 20–40 U/kg but consumed significantly less factor 1,828 versus 2,900 U/kg/year [26]. In a 6-year longitudinal study patients on >45 weeks of prophylaxis per year had significantly ($p < 0.00001$) lower Pettersson scores than those not on prophylaxis [18]. In a prospective study of long-term secondary prophylaxis, radiographic changes stabilized in 10/16 joints and worsened in 6/16 [42].

Barriers

Despite currently being the best option to reduce bleeding rates in persons with hemophilia, many barriers to prophylaxis exist and some patients experience complications related to regular factor delivery. The utilization of prophylactic therapy varies widely even between some developed countries. For example, the frequency of prophylaxis use among patients with severe hemophilia A in Canada is 77 versus 47% in the Unites States [48]. The first barrier to good care is that many persons with bleeding disorders in developing countries lack access to a diagnosis of their bleeding disorder. If these patients are fortunate enough to have an accurate diagnosis the lack of access to safe clotting factor concentrates is the biggest barrier to treatment. It is estimated that 80% of persons with hemophilia worldwide live in developing countries and have no or limited access to safe factor products [49]. If a virally safe product exists, the expense of long-term prophylaxis is the next barrier that patients face [50]. It requires significantly more factor usage than intermittent/demand therapy [28, 51]. In some developed countries even when abundant factor is available, many patients are not on long-term prophylaxis [52, 53]. Compliance with frequent injections, particularly in young children, requires a compliant patient and a dedicated family [54]. One small study suggests that the use of low-volume factor decreases the need for more than one intravenous stick and is preferred by both families and nursing staff [55]. Some patients typically younger children will require a venous access device to deliver such frequent infusions due to lack of peripheral access. First the device must be implanted surgically and the patient risks anesthesia and bleeding. Mechanical complications such as leakage and extrusion sometimes occur [56]. These devices are also associated with an increased risk of infection and thrombosis. Rates of infection vary from 0.14 to 3.4 infections/1,000 catheter days [56–63]. CVADs placed for immune tolerance have higher rates of infection than those placed for prophylaxis [56, 57, 60, 63]. A growing body of literature suggests that rates of thrombosis in hemophilia patients with CVADs are quite high. Eight of 15 (53%) patients with central venous devices that were studied by venography had evidence of thrombosis [64]. Of note, only 5 of these patients had clinical evidence of thrombosis. A recent prospective study of CVAD thrombosis revealed that 81% of patients had radiological evidence of thrombosis at a median of 6.4 years after catheter placement [65].

Discontinuation of Prophylaxis

Many patients interrupt their prophylactic schedules intermittently and some discontinue permanently. Little is currently understood about the clinical relevance of discontinuation of prophylaxis. In vitro data suggests that articular cartilage of young animals is more susceptible to blood-induced joint damage than more mature cartilage [66]. The Dutch experience recently compared the radiographic results between patients who continued on primary prophylaxis and those who discontinued prophylaxis [67]. The median age at discontinuation of prophylaxis was 20.4 years. The median number of joint bleeds and the median Pettersson score were actually higher in patients who had never stopped prophylaxis. These differences, however, did not achieve statistical significance. As radiographic progression is a slow process, this may be related to a relatively shorter follow-up for radiographs in the discontinuation group. Additionally, those patients who permanently discontinued prophylaxis tended to have a milder bleeding pattern than those who continued prophylaxis. Further data and long-term studies are needed to see if a group of patients who can safely discontinue prophylaxis can be identified.

Conclusion

In countries that have access to adequate amounts of safe factor products, prevention of bleeds and the morbidity caused by bleeding episodes should be the goal of care. Prophylactic factor usage should be individualized based upon patient characteristics, family situation, frequency and location of bleeding, pharmacokinetic response to factor, venous access, patient lifestyle and economic impact. The safest product should be utilized in the most economically responsible manner. Unresolved issues which will only be answered by long-term cooperative trials include when to start prophylaxis, appropriate joint imaging techniques, appropriate functional joint health scoring, and whether prophylaxis can be discontinued safely. Adverse events such as the risk of inhibitor development, complications related to CVADs and impact of treatment regimen on quality of life should be carefully considered. Techniques to avoid placement of CVADs should be explored. Methods to reduce the rates of infection and thrombosis associated with these lines should be investigated. Treatment centers should continue to work together to optimize prophylaxis regimens and to standardize and validate outcome measures. The community should continue to support basic and translational research into the pathophysiology of joint disease, inhibitor development and factor antigenicity and immunogenicity. Developing products with longer half-lives or alternate routes of delivery also need further research. Developing countries should continue investigating minimal treatment strategies to manage the progression of joint disease. With a relatively rare disease such as hemophilia, communication and cooperation between treatment centers is the best way to improve care for all patients with bleeding disorders.

References

1 Mannucci PM, Tuddenham EGD: Medical progress; the hemophilias – from royal genes to gene therapy. N Engl J Med 2001;344:1773–1779.
2 Mannucci PM, Tuddenbam EGD: The hemophilias: progress and problems. Semin Hematol 1999;36(suppl 7):104–117.
3 Nilsson IM, Hedner U, Ahlberg A: Haemophilia prophylaxis in Sweden. Acta Paediatr Scand 1976;63:129–135.
4 Rosner F: Hemophilia in the Talmud and rabbinic writings. Ann Intern Med 1969;70:833–837.
5 Otto JC: An account of an hemorrhagic disposition existing in certain families. Med Repos 1803;6:1–9.
6 Pavlovsky A: Contribution to the pathogenesis of hemophilia. Blood 1947;2:185.
7 Biggs R, Douglas AS, Macfarlane RG, Dacie JV, Pitney WR, Merskey PMID: Christmas disease: a condition previously mistaken for haemophilia. Br Med J 1952;ii:1378–1382.
8 Farr AD: Treatment of haemophilia by transfusion: the first recorded case. J R Soc Med 1981;74:301–305.
9 Davie ER: A brief historical review of the waterfall/cascade of blood coagulation. J Biol Chem 2003;278:50819–50832.
10 Pool JG, Hershgold EJ, Pappenhagen AR: High potency antihaemophiliac factor concentrate prepared from cryoglobulin precipitate. Nature 1964;203:312.
11 Hann I, Abshire T, Lusher J, Recht M, Mathew P, Gorelick K, Charnigo R; ReFactor AF Study Group: Interim analysis of the clinic evaluation of refacto AF, a B-domain deleted recombinant FVIII (BDDrFVIII), manufactured by a novel albumin- and monoclonal antibody-free process (abstract 173). Blood 2003;102: 815a.
12 Recht M, Abshire T, Lusher J, Manco-Johnson M, Gorelick K, Daly S; ReFactor AF Study Group: Results of a single-dose, randomized, double-blind, 2-period crossover pharmacokinetic study of B-domain deleted recombinant FVIII (BDDrFVIII), current manufacturing process (ReFacto), and BDDrFVIII, albumin-free manufacturing process (ReFacto AF) (abstract 2942). Blood 2003;102:53a.
13 Ewenstein B, Collins P, Shapiro A, Tarantino M, Blanchette V, Rogy S; rAHF-PFM Study Group: Global evaluation of ADVATE rAHF-PFM, an advanced category antihemophilic factor prepared using a plasma/albumin-free method. Blood 2003;102:172.
14 Hoots WK, Blanchette V, Shapiro A, Navales L, Spotts G, Togy S, Ewenstein B: Clinical evaluation of an advanced category recombinant FVIII, anti-hemophilic factor (recombinant) plasma/albumin-free method (rAHF-PFM) in pediatric previously treated patients (PTPs). J Thromb Haemost 2003;164:2.
15 MASAC Recommendation #117. MASAC Recommendation Concerning Prophylaxis (Prophylactic Administration of Clotting Factor Concentrate to Prevent Bleeding). National Hemophilia Foundation, June 9, 2001.
16 Brown SA, Aledor LM; Round Table Group: Unresolved issues in prophylaxis. Haemophilia 2002;8:817–821.
17 Nilsson IM, Berntorp E, Lofqvist T, Pettersson H: Twenty-five years' experience of prophylactic treatment in severe haemophilia A and B. J Intern Med 1992;232:25–32.

18 Aledort LM, Haschmeyer RH, Pettersson H; Orthopaedic Outcome Study Group: A longitudinal study of orthopaedic outcomes for severe factor VIII deficient haemophiliacs. J Intern Med 1994;236:391–399.
19 Astermark J, Petrini P, Tengborn L, Schulman S, Ljung R, Berntorp E: Primary prophylaxis in severe haemophilia should be started at an early age but can be individualized. Br J Haematol 1999;105:1109–1113.
20 Miners AH, Sabin CA, Tolley KH, Lee CA: Primary prophylaxis for individuals with severe haemophilia: how many hospital visits could treatment prevent? J Intern Med 2000; 247:493–499.
21 Fischer K, Van Der Bom JG, Mauser-Bunschoten EP, Roosendaal G, Prejs R, De Kleijn P, Grobbee DE, Van Den Berg M: The effects of postponing prophylactic treatment on long-term outcome in patients with severe hemophilia. Blood 2002;99:2337–2341.
22 Schramm W: Experience with prophylaxis in Germany. Semin Hematol 1993;30(suppl 2): 12–15.
23 Van Dijk K, Fischer K, Van Der Bom JG, Mauser-Bunschoten EP, Roosendaal GK, Van Den Berg HM: Variability in bleeding pattern of severe hemophilia. Blood 2004;104:abstract 3094.
24 Ettingshausen CE, Zyschka A, Saguer IM, Heller C, Klingebiel T, Kreuz W: The role of age at first exposure and therapy regimen on the development of neutralizing FVIII antibodies in hemophilia A. Blood 2004;104: abstract 3082.
25 Santagostino E, Rocino A, Mancuso ME, Mazzucconi MG, Mancuso G, Messina M, Tagliaferri A, Luciani M, Boeri E, Mannucci PM: Impact of early factor VIII exposure, prophylaxis and prenatal/perinatal events on inhibitor risk in children with hemophilia A: a case-control study. Blood 2004;104:abstract 37.
26 Van Den Berg HM, Fischer K, Mauser-Bunschoten EP, Beek FJA, Roosendaal G, Van Der Bom JG, Nieuwenhuis HK: Long-term outcome of individualized prophylactic treatment of children with severe haemophilia. Br J Haematol 2001;112:561–565.
27 Van Dijk K, Van Der Bom JG, Bax KMA, Van Der Zee DC, Van Den Berg HM: Use of implantable venous access devices in children with severe hemophilia: benefits and burden. Haematologica 2004;89:189–194.
28 Smith PS, Teutsch SM, Shaffer PA, Rolka H, Evatt B: Episodic versus prophylactic infusions for hemophilia A: a cost-effectiveness analysis. J Pediatr 1996;129:424–431.
29 Fischer K, Van Der Bom JG, Molho P, Negrier C, Mauseer-Bunschoten EP, Roosendaal G, De Kleijn P, Groggee DE, Van Den Berg HM: Prophylactic versus on-demand treatment strategies for severe haemophilia: a comparison of costs and long-term outcome. Haemophilia 2002;8:745–752.
30 Brackmann HH, Eickhoff HJ, Oldenburg J, Hammerstein U: Long-term therapy and on-demand treatment of children and adolescents with severe haemophilia A: 12 years of experience. Haemostasis 1992;22:251–258.
31 Steen Carlsson K, Hojgard S, Glomstein A, Lethagen S, Schulman S, Tengborn L, Lindgren A, Berntorp E, Lindgren B: On-demand vs. prophylactic treatment for severe haemophilia in Norway and Sweden: differences in treatment characteristics and outcome. Haemophilia 2003;9:555–566.
32 Gringeri A: Long-term aspects of hemophilia B treatment. Part II. Blood Coagul Fibrinolysis 2004;15(suppl 2):S15–S16.
33 Fischer K, Astermark J, Van Der Bom JG, Ljung R, Berntorp E: Prophylactic treatment for severe haemophilia: Comparison of an intermediate-dose to a high-dose regimen. Haemophilia 2002;8:753–760.
34 Fischer K, Van Den Berg M: Prophylaxis for severe haemophilia: clinical and economical issues. Haemophilia 2003;9:376–381.
35 Bjorkman S, Berntorp E: Pharmacokinetics of coagulation factors clinical relevance for patients with haemophilia. Clin Pharmacokinet 2001;40:815–832.
36 Blanchette V, Shapiro AD, Liesner R, Hernandez F, Retzios AD, Schroth P, Fritsch S, Spotts G, Ewenstein BM: Characterization of the pharmacokinetics of rFVIII in young preschool children with hemophilia, including an analysis of the influence of age and body weight. Blood 2004;104:abstract 3084.
37 Carlsson M, Berntorp E, Bjorkman S, Lethagen S, Ljung R: Improving cost-effectiveness by pharmacokinetic dosing of factor VIII in prophylactic treatment of haemophilia A. Haemophilia 1997;3:96–101.
38 Blanchette VS, Rivard GE, Israels SJ, Robinson KS, Babyn PS, McLimont MJ, Hilliard PE, Feldman BM: Musculoskeletal results from the Canadian hemophilia dose-escalation prophylaxis trial; in Abstracts of the American Society of Hematology 45th Annual Meeting and Exposition, San Diego, Calif. 2003, p 171.
39 Kreuz W, Escuriola-Ettingshausen C, Funk M, Schmidt H, Kornhuber B: When should prophylactic treatment in patients with haemophilia A and B start? – The German experience. Haemophilia 1998;4:413–417.
40 Petrini P, Lindvall N, Egberg N, Blomback M: Prophylaxis with factor concentrates in preventing hemophilic arthropathy. Am J Pediatr Hematol Oncol 1991;13:280–287.
41 Leisner RJ, Khair K, Hann IM: The impact of prophylactic treatment on children with severe haemophilia. Br J Haematol 1996;92:973–978.
42 Manco-Johnson MJ, Nuss R, Geraghty S, Funk S, Kilcoyne R: Results of secondary prophylaxis in children with severe hemophilia. Am J Hematol 1994 47:113–117.
43 Arnold WD, Hilgartner MW: Hemophilic arthopathy. J Bone Joint Surg Am 1977;59:287–305.
44 Pettersson H, Ahlberg A, Nilsson IM: A radiologic classification of hemophilic arthropathy. Clin Orthop 1980;149:153–159.
45 Nuss R, Kilcoyne F, Geraghty S, Shroyer ALW, Rosky JW, Mawhinney S, Wiedel J, Manco-Johnson M: MRI findings in haemophilic joints treated with radiosynoviorthesis with development of an MRI scale of joint damage. Haemophilia 2000;6:162–169.
46 Kilcoyne RF, Nuss R: Radiological assessment of haemophilic arthropathy with emphasis on MRI findings. Haemophilia 2003;9(suppl 1): 57–64.
47 Lundin B, Pettersson H, Ljung R: A new magnetic resonance imaging scoring method for assessment of haemophilic arthropathy. Haemophilia 2004;10:383–389.
48 Blanchette VS, Mccready M, Achonu C, Abdolell M, Rivard G, Manco-Johnson MJ: A survey of factor prophylaxis in boys with haemophilia followed in North American haemophilia treatment centers. Haemophilia 2003; 9(suppl 1):19–26.
49 Srivastava A: Choice of factor concentrates for haemophilia: a developing world perspective. Haemophilia 2001;7:117–122.
50 Tussell J, Perez-Bianco R: Prophylaxis in developed and in emerging countries. Haemophilia 2002;8:183–188.
51 Panicker J, Warrier I, Thomas R, Lusher JM: The overall effectiveness of prophylaxis in severe haemophilia. Haemophilia 2003;9:272–278.
52 Shapiro AD: Why is primary prophylaxis underutilized in the United States? Haemophilia 2003;9:670–672.
53 Butler RB, McClure W, Wulff K: Practice patterns in haemophilia A therapy – a survey of treatment centres in the United States. Haemophilia 2003;9:549–554.
54 Hacker MR, Geraghty S, Manco-Johnson M: Barriers to compliance with prophylaxis therapy in haemophilia. Haemophilia 2001;7:392–396.
55 Butler RB: Clinical convenience of low volume FVIII infusions in pediatric hemophilia patients. Hemaware 2004;10:114.
56 Bollard CM, Teague LR, Berry EW, Ockelford PA: The use of central venous catheters (portacaths) in children with haemophilia. Haemophilia 2000;6:66–70.
57 Ljung R, van den Berg M, Petrini P, Tengborn L, Scheibel E, Kekomaki R, Effenberger W: Port-a-cath usage in children with haemophilia: experience of 53 cases. Acta Paediatr 2004; 87:1051–1054.
58 Perkins JL, Johnson VA, Osip JM, Christie BA, Nelson SC, Moertel CL, Heisel MA: The use of implantable venous access devices (IVADs) in children with hemophilia. J Pediatr Hematol Oncol 1997;19:339–344.
59 Miller K, Buchanan GR, Zappa S, Cochran C, Laufenberg J, Medeiros D, Sanders J: Implantable venous access devices in children with hemophilia: a report of low infection rates. J Pediatr 1998;132:934–938.

60 Liesner RJ, Vora AJ, Hann IM, Lilleymann JS: Use of central venous catheters in children with severe congenital coagulopathy. Br J Haematol 1995;91:203–207.
61 Srivaths PR, Rozans MK, Kelly E, Venkateswaran L: *Bacillus cereus* central line infection in an immunocompetent child with hemophilia. J Pediatr Hematol Oncol 2004;26: 194–196.
62 Santagostino E, Gringeri A, Muca-Perja M, Mannucci PM: A prospective clinical trial of implantable central venous access in children with haemophilia. Br J Haematol 1998;102: 1224–1228.
63 Valentino LA, Ewenstein B, Navickis RJ, Wilkes MM: Central venous access devices in haemophilia. Haemophilia 2004;10:134–146.
64 Journeycake JM, Quinn CT, Miller KL, Zajac JL, Buchanan GR: Catheter-related deep venous thrombosis in children with hemophilia. Blood 2001;98:1727–1731.
65 Price VE, Carcao M, Connolly B, Chait P, Daneman A, Temple M, Stain AM, Sung L, Al-Tralbbosi H, Blanchette VS: A prospective, longitudinal study of central venous catheter-related deep venous thrombosis in boys with hemophilia. J Thromb Haemost 2004;2:737–742.
66 Hooiveld MJ, Roosendaal G, Vianen ME, van den Berg HM, Bijlsma JW, Lafeber FP: Immature articular cartilage is more susceptible to blood-induced damage than mature articular cartilage: an in vivo animal study. Arthritis Rheum 2003;48:396–403.
67 Fischer K, Van Der Bom JG, Prejs R, Mauser-Bunschoten EP, Roosendaal G, Grobbee DE, Van Den Berg HM: Discontinuation of prophylactic therapy in severe haemophilia: incidence and effects of outcome. Haemophilia 2001;7:544–550.

Acta Haematologica

Acta Haematol 2006;115:172–179
DOI: 10.1159/000090931

New Approaches in the Management of Inhibitor Patients

Guy Young

Children's Hospital of Orange County, Orange, Calif., USA

Key Words
Hemophilia · Inhibitors

Abstract
The most serious current complication of factor replacement therapy for hemophilia patients is the development of neutralizing antibodies to the factor termed inhibitors. Patients with high-titer inhibitors frequently develop serious bleeding complications which do not respond to standard factor replacement therapy. Therefore, they must be treated with the so-called bypassing agents, recombinant factor VIIa and activated prothrombin complex concentrates, neither of which is as effective as standard factor replacement in patients without inhibitors. Immune tolerance therapy aimed at eradicating inhibitors is successful in a majority of patients; however, a sizable minority will have life-long inhibitors and often develop debilitating joint disease. The ultimate goal is to develop strategies aimed at preventing inhibitor development though these have not been realized yet. Until this is achieved, additional novel approaches are needed to improve the treatment of bleeding episodes and to better treat arthropathy once it develops. Finally, there is no laboratory monitoring device which can predict the clinical response of patients to bypassing agents. Thus another goal of current research is to develop such a tool which will enable the individualization of bypassing agent.

Introduction

The most serious complication of hemophilia resulting from the use of factor concentrates is the development of neutralizing antibodies known as inhibitors. Such inhibitors preclude (in many patients) the use of standard and effective factor concentrates resulting in more bleeding complications [1]. While most inhibitors are either transient or resolve with immune tolerance therapy, approximately 15% of factor VIII (FVIII)-deficient patients and 3% of factor IX (FIX)-deficient patients have persistent clinically significant inhibitors which result in severe morbidity [2]. This particular complication of therapy is the most serious concern in managing patients with hemophilia in the current era and has spurred research into methods to reduce inhibitor development, improve methods to eradicate inhibitors once they develop, better treat bleeding episodes and arthropathy, and develop an effective laboratory monitoring device for bypass therapy.

Prevention of Inhibitor Development

A major goal for the management of hemophilia is to reduce the incidence of inhibitor development. Thus far, all of the new recombinant FVIII products have demonstrated a similar incidence of inhibitor formation of around 30% [1]. Although some of these inhibitors are transient, many patients require expensive and inconvenient immune tolerance therapy which though successful

KARGER
Fax +41 61 306 12 34
E-Mail karger@karger.ch
www.karger.com

0001–5792/06/1154–0172$23.50/0

Accessible online at:
www.karger.com/aha

Guy Young, MD
Children's Hospital of Orange County
455 S. Main Street
Orange, CA 92868 (USA)
Tel. +1 714 532 8459, Fax +1 714 532 8771, E-Mail gyoung@choc.org

in ~70% of patients requires large amounts of frequently administered factor for many months and occasionally years [3]. One approach to prevent inhibitors is to bioengineer less immunogenic factor replacement products. Peter Lollar at Emory University has pioneered methods of reducing FVIII immunogenicity by altering the amino acid sequence of FVIII thereby removing the 'immunogenic' portions of the molecule without a reduction in the function of the protein [4]. Other approaches at preventing inhibitor formation include delaying the use of factor concentrates [5], administering factor concentrates with immune-suppressing medication [6, 7], and even early introduction of factor concentrates [8]. A few small studies have demonstrated that inhibitor development is more common in patients who receive large amounts of factor concentrates early in life [9]. If such data are confirmed in additional studies, delaying the use of factor concentrates may be one way to prevent inhibitors, and could be considered in patients at especially high risk such as those with mutations that predispose to inhibitors and those with a family history of inhibitors, for example. If such patients bleed, the use of alternative agents such as recombinant factor VIIa (rFVIIa) could be employed to achieve hemostasis until the age at which standard factor replacement would not likely lead to inhibitor formation. This approach would need to be balanced with the potential benefits of early prophylaxis. Experiments in mice whereby factor concentrates were administered concomitantly with anti-CD40 ligand [6] or anti-CTLA4 [7] (to block the B7-CD28 pathway) nearly eliminated inhibitor development; however, studies in humans did not demonstrate a prolonged benefit [10]. Additional studies in animals have demonstrated that induction of tolerance via factor infusions on day of life 0 is effective at preventing inhibitor formation [8]. While the above data is intriguing, further studies are needed to determine the best methods to prevent inhibitor formation, and this should remain a focus in hemophilia research until substantial reductions in inhibitor formation are achieved.

Immune Tolerance Therapy

A second goal of current research in inhibitor patients is to improve the outcome and reduce the cost and inconvenience of immune tolerance therapy. At this time, there are several therapeutic regimens for immune tolerance induction ranging from low doses of factor given every other day to much larger doses given daily and regimens that incorporate immunosuppressive therapy along with factor infusions (Malmo regimen) [3]. (Most of this data and the subsequent discussion below is limited to FVIII deficiency. Inhibitors to FIX are less common and there is a paucity of data from which to make recommendations for the management of FIX inhibitors.) Unfortunately, these trials lacked uniform criteria for patient eligibility and were not controlled leading to a lack of consensus on the best approach. Currently, the International Immune Tolerance Study under the direction of Donna DiMichele and Charles Hay is actively recruiting patients from many countries. This study is randomizing patients to 50 units/kg every other day versus 100 units/kg daily. Hopefully this study will determine the most efficacious and cost-effective approach for the eradication of inhibitors. Although immune tolerance therapy as described is the only established treatment for the eradication of inhibitors, there are other approaches being considered. There are several reports describing the achievement of tolerance utilizing an FVIII product which contains von Willebrand factor in patients who had previously failed to achieve tolerance with pure FVIII concentrates [11]. The mechanism for this response is unknown but undoubtedly involves von Willebrand factor in some way. Further studies are indicated not only in patients in whom immune tolerance failed with recombinant FVIII but also as a first-line approach. Alternatively, a recent report of 2 cases (one FVIII and one FIX deficiency) demonstrated the use of the anti-CD20 antibody rituximab for the eradication of hemophilia inhibitors in patients that did not respond to conventional immune tolerance therapy. The patient with the FVIII inhibitor had resolution of the inhibitor with a follow-up of 11 months; however, the therapy failed for a patient with an FIX inhibitor [12]. Such therapy is effective in a number of autoimmune diseases; however, the nature of the antibodies in inhibitor patients is different as these are 'naturally' occurring alloantibodies arising from an appropriate immune response to a 'foreign' protein as opposed to a loss of tolerance to self-antigens as is the case in autoimmune disease. While this approach is intriguing, controlled studies will need to be performed in order to deem such therapy appropriate especially as a first-line treatment. In addition to the above currently available approaches, there are some novel approaches which may offer improvements in the future. One such approach is aimed at reducing the neutralizing effect of the inhibitory antibody rather than eradicating it by using peptide decoys which mimic the binding site of the epitope on FVIII [13]. In theory, this approach may allow inhibitor patients to be treated with replacement FVIII as in noninhibitor patients.

Table 1. Currently available concentrates for inhibitor patients

Factor concentrate	Pros	Cons	Comments
PCCs	Relatively inexpensive	Not as effective as APCCs Potentially thrombogenic	APCCs have largely supplanted the use of PCCs in inhibitor patients
APCCs (FEIBA)	Long history of use Long half-life relative to rFVIIa Efficacy of 80–90% in clinical trials More effective than PCC	Potentially thrombogenic (mostly demonstrated in older publications) No measurable laboratory parameter Plasma-derived Presence of FVIII potentially leading to anamnesis of inhibitor	Recent data suggest the risk of thrombotic complications with standard doses is low
rFVIIa	Recombinant product with no requirement for human plasma proteins in production Efficacy of ~90% with about 2 doses in clinical trials Low rate of thrombotic complications	Short half-life leading to the need for multiple daily doses Efficacy in clinical trials does not seem to translate to clinical practice Most effective dosing regimen is unknown No measurable laboratory parameter	2 current clinical trials are assessing rFVIIa versus FEIBA and 1 is assessing 2 dosing regimens for rFVIIa A few reports describe thromboelastography and thrombin generation assays as an effective laboratory parameter

PCC = Prothrombin complex concentrates.

Treatment of Bleeding Episodes

Another important goal for inhibitor patients is to improve the management of bleeding symptoms and to prevent chronic joint disease. The management of bleeding episodes in inhibitor patients depends on the patient's inhibitor titer as well as whether the inhibitor is a low or high responder. Other important factors to consider when selecting the best hemostatic therapy for each bleed in a given patient include the severity and location of the bleed as well as the availability of specific therapies and the patient's previous response to specific therapies. For example, a low-titer, low-responder patient with a simple hemarthrosis can be treated with standard factor replacement albeit at higher doses. For patients with high-titer inhibitors, however, standard factor replacement is generally not effective. At present, there are only 2 hemostatic agents available for the management of bleeding in patients with high-titer inhibitors (table 1). These are activated prothrombin complex concentrates [(APCC), factor eight inhibitor bypass activity (FEIBA), Baxter, Glendale, Calif., USA] and rFVIIa (Novoseven, Bagsvaerd, Denmark). Previously porcine FVIII was another option; however, it is currently no longer available, and while prothrombin complex concentrates are still available, they have been supplanted by APCC for the management of bleeding in inhibitor patients. While both APCC and rFVIIa demonstrate excellent efficacy in clinical trials (around 90%) [14, 15], the actual clinical efficacy is less than that reported in clinical trials in the opinion of many treaters. Furthermore, some patients do not respond well to either therapy and develop significant bleeding complications and chronic joint disease. There are currently 2 clinical trials aimed at establishing the efficacy of the 2 agents in comparative trials. In addition, one of these trials is also testing the hypothesis that a single higher dose (270 μg/kg) of rFVIIa is more effective than the currently approved dosing (90 μg/kg for 3 doses) with a placebo-controlled double-blind method. The results of these studies should be available in the next year. Data from uncontrolled trials suggest that higher doses of rFVIIa (200–300 μg/kg/dose) are more effective than the currently approved dose range (90–120 μg/kg/dose) [16, 17].

Another recently published approach for bleeds that are refractory to either agent alone is to use sequential therapy with both FEIBA and rFVIIa. One study demonstrated improvement in the ACT in inhibitor patients treated with FEIBA for whom rFVIIa was added ex vivo [18]. Furthermore, a report on the use of sequential ther-

Table 2. Current and future improvements for inhibitor patients (see table 3 for methods to prevent inhibitor formation)

Shortcoming	Technique	Current availability	Comments/future availability
Ineffective (less effective than standard factor) hemostasis with currently available agents	Use agents (APCC and rFVIIa) in combination	yes	Small case series demonstrated safety and suggested efficacy
Few available effective agents	Develop new agents	no	Recombinant porcine FVIII (OBI-1) in clinical trials (potentially available in next few years)
Current agents with short half-life (rFVIIa) or plasma-derived with history of thrombogenicity (APCC)	Bioengineer rFVIIa to have a longer half-life Use rFVIIa in combination with FX for prolonged effect with less thrombogenicity than APCC	no	Novel superactive rFVIIa molecules are in preclinical testing Early evidence of the synergistic effect of rFVIIa and FX
Inability to prevent bleeding episodes	Use rFVIIa or APCC prophylactically	yes	Limited evidence demonstrating efficacy in a few patients Clinical trial of prophylactic rFVIIa and prophylactic FEIBA are under way
Inability to eradicate inhibitors in all patients	Improve immune tolerance therapy with factor	yes	International clinical trial underway
	Use novel currently available agents	yes	Case report of resolution with rituximab

apy with APCC and rFVIIa demonstrated the safety of this approach and suggested efficacy in 91 patient-days of therapy with no patient demonstrating clinical or laboratory evidence of thrombosis or disseminated intravascular coagulopathy [19].

Prophylaxis in Inhibitor Patients

Besides therapy aimed at treating bleeding episodes once they occur, there are several small reports which describe the use of APCC or rFVIIa for prophylaxis of bleeding in inhibitor patients. Such therapy has been advocated for particularly difficult patients who develop either multiple, significant bleeding episodes or target joints. Data for the prophylactic use of FEIBA from a small uncontrolled trial demonstrated improvement in arthropathy in 2 of 7 patients leading to their ability to return to school [20]. There are 2 reports describing the use of rFVIIa given in a prophylactic mode. Combined, the 2 reports describe the treatment of 3 patients (2 with target joints and 1 with multiple severe bleeding episodes) with resolution of the target joints and reduction in severe bleeding episodes and reduced hospitalizations [21, 22]. A clinical trial evaluating the safety and efficacy of rFVIIa given once daily at a dose of either 90 or 270 μg/kg (in a blinded fashion) is under way. There is also a current study evaluating the utility of FEIBA for prophylaxis in inhibitor patients. While there is no doubt about the efficacy of prophylactic factor replacement in noninhibitor patients, there are as yet no firm data supporting the use of prophylaxis in inhibitor patients. It is the author's opinion that prophylaxis for inhibitor patients with either APCC or rFVIIa should only be considered for the most severely affected patients such as those with recurrent life- or limb-threatening bleeds or those in whom target joints develop for whom other approaches such as synovectomy are not feasible.

Novel Hemostatic Agents

Despite the reasonable efficacy of FEIBA and rFVIIa, novel hemostatic therapies for inhibitor patients with improved efficacy and safety are warranted. One approach involves the bioengineering of rFVIIa to improve its biologic profile by enhancing thrombin generation [23]. Another group has demonstrated both in vitro and in vivo (in a monkey model) that combining plasma-derived

Table 3. Adjunctive therapy for joint disease

Agent/technique	Pros	Cons	Availability
Radioisotopic synovectomy	Minimally invasive	Risks of radiation	In select centers
Arthroscopic synovectomy	Effects last longer than radioisotopic synovectomy	Invasive procedure with significant bleeding risks	Available in most centers
Novel anti-inflammatory/ antiangiogenic agents (COX-2 inhibitors)	Oral No effect on platelet function Much less risky than surgery	Study demonstrating safety and potential efficacy in 28 patients [27]	1 available agent (celecoxib) Cardiovascular complications noted in cancer prevention trials are less concerning in hemophilia due to the lower risk of cardiovascular disease and the manner in which these agents were used in the cancer prevention trials (high daily dose for extended periods of time)

FVIIa with plasma-derived FX resulted in a longer duration of thrombin generation as compared to rFVIIa alone but without the thrombogenicity of APCC [24]. Preclinical studies are ongoing in the development of these agents. Another approach is to improve the safety and availability of porcine FVIII by developing recombinant porcine FVIII [25]. A clinical trial of this agent termed OBI-1 is underway (see table 2 for current and future developments in inhibitor patients).

Adjunctive Therapy for Joint Disease

Preventing joint disease via regular factor infusions and close follow-up of joint examinations by skilled personnel is of paramount importance in the management of hemophilia. For patients who develop recurrent joint bleeds (target joints), the institution of regular factor infusions if not already in place is critical if chronic joint disease is to be prevented; however, as discussed above, this is not as effective (if effective at all) for inhibitor patients. Aside from factor replacement therapy and physical therapy when appropriate, there are some novel approaches that merit consideration (table 3). Since recurrent joint hemorrhage leads to inflammation and angiogenesis resulting in synovial hypertrophy which can lead to more bleeding and eventual permanent joint destruction, agents with anti-inflammatory and antiangiogenic properties may be efficacious. Unfortunately the standard nonsteroidal anti-inflammatory agents affect platelet function and are, therefore, relatively contraindicated in patients with bleeding disorders. Newer agents known as cyclooxygenase-2 (COX-2) inhibitors maintain the anti-inflammatory properties of NSAIDS, however do not affect platelet function. Furthermore, these agents have antiangiogenic properties not inherent to NSAIDS and may provide further benefit by reducing the formation of new friable blood vessels. A case report described the use of a COX-2 inhibitor in an adult hemophilia patient with chronic synovitis which the patient was treating with multiple doses of factor [26]. Treatment with daily rofecoxib significantly reduced factor usage implying improvement in this patient's synovitis. We recently completed a review of the use of rofecoxib in 28 adults and children for treatment of acute joint bleeding (along with factor), for treatment of target joints (with factor prophylaxis), and for chronic synovitis/arthritis and pain. There were no adverse events noted directly attributed to rofecoxib, and there was the suggestion of efficacy for all four indications [27]. Unfortunately, rofecoxib was recently linked to an increase in cardiovascular events in patients on high-dose long-term use during a cancer prevention trial leading to its voluntary withdrawal from the market by its manufacturer (www.merck.com/newsroom/press_release/product/2004_0930.html). We believe patients with hemophilia who are considered at relatively low risk for cardiovascular disease [28, 29] and who could benefit from improved joint function and reduced pain are patients in whom the benefit to risk ratio of COX-2 inhibitors is favorable. Patients with improved joint function and less pain are likely to exercise more, thus mitigating the increased risk for cardiovascular disease. Furthermore, celecoxib has not been linked thus far with cardiovascular disease [30, 31]. Clearly, additional studies including randomized, placebo-controlled trials are indicated to assess the safety and efficacy of COX-2 inhibitors before widespread use can be recommended. We do feel, however, that inhibitor patients with target joints should have a trial of COX-2 inhibitors prior to undergoing more risky surgical approaches (see below).

Another mode of therapy which though not novel has been used more extensively for hemophilia patients in recent years is radioisotopic synovectomy [32]. This procedure entails the injection of a radioisotope (usually ^{32}P) into the affected joint with the goal of destroying the hypertrophied synovial tissue and preventing its reaccumulation. This treatment is currently indicated for patients with target joints who do not respond to factor prophylaxis and is in lieu of more invasive arthroscopic and open surgical synovectomies which are particularly risky in inhibitor patients. This treatment approach has had an overall high rate of success with minimal complications. A concern with this approach as with all radiation therapy is the potential for development of malignancy. There are 2 reported cases of malignancy in hemophilia patients in whom this procedure was performed (pers. commun.); however, it is not clear whether this represents a higher than expected rate of malignancy based on the known incidence or whether the malignancies are related to the radiation. It is imperative all patients who have undergone radioisotopic synovectomies have long-term follow-up in order to determine the true rate of carcinogenicity.

Laboratory Monitoring

The clinical response to standard factor replacement is correlated reasonably well with the level of factor achieved after an infusion of factor. This along with the knowledge of the pharmacokinetics of standard factor concentrates has led to the development of treatment guidelines for the management of bleeding episodes and for the prevention of surgical bleeding [33]. Since inhibitor patients must be treated with bypassing agents, the same strategy does not apply except for patients with low-titer inhibitors who are being managed with standard factor replacement. At present, there is no laboratory method which correlates with the clinical response of bypassing agents. Although one can assay the prothrombin time, activated partial thromboplastin time, FVII and FVIIa levels, these do not in general correlate with the clinical response. Novel methods are needed which can predict the clinical response from a dose of APCC or rFVIIa. Several devices have emerged as potential candidates for such monitoring, and the reader is referred to the review by Key and Nelsestuen [34] for details. The leading candidates at this point are thromboelastography (TEG) and the thrombin generation test. The advantages of TEG are the fact that it utilizes whole blood (plasma can be used as well), can be done rapidly, is easy to transport for point-of-service testing in the clinic, is relatively inexpensive, and is simple to use. The advantages of the thrombin generation test include its ability to quantify thrombin generation more accurately. A few reports have demonstrated the utility of TEG to determine the effectiveness of rFVIIa and APCC either in inhibitor patients ex vivo and in vivo [35, 36]. Furthermore, the in vivo study also demonstrated the ability to monitor sequential therapy with rFVIIa and APCC that was previously described. Both methods are currently under further investigation as potential laboratory monitoring devices for bypassing agents in inhibitor patients. Other methods under exploration include the clot signature analyzer, platelet contractile force, and modified activated clotting time [34].

Conclusion

There have been significant improvements in the prognosis of hemophilia over the past decade; however, in the minority of patients with inhibitors, there remain significant obstacles to achieving the same degree of quality of life enjoyed by most noninhibitor patients. Thus novel approaches and technologies are necessary in order to improve the quality of life in inhibitor patients. Ideally, prevention of inhibitors altogether will obviate the need for any other therapies; however, this goal does not appear to be possible in the near future. Improvements in eradicating inhibitors may be realized sooner with either improved immune tolerance therapy or with new immunomodulatory agents such as rituximab or others. Additionally, there is a need to evaluate in more detail the use of FVIII/VWF concentrates as being potentially more effective at eradicating inhibitors than recombinant concentrates. The management of bleeding episodes is evolving and may include combination therapy with rFVIIa and APCC which is currently available or combination therapy with rFVIIa and other concentrates such as FX which may become available in the future. Other novel approaches involve the bioengineering of rFVIIa to generate molecules with increased thrombin generation or longer duration of action. Such novel hemostatic approaches will require a laboratory correlate and investigations are ongoing to identify laboratory tests that will correlate with the clinical efficacy of these agents. Finally, for patients with established joint disease, improved therapy to maximize joint outcome needs further investigation. These may include anti-inflammatory and antiangiogenic agents such as COX-2 inhibitors or others and improved surgical techniques to treat hemophilic arthropathy which occurs in many inhibitor patients. The gains made in the management of noninhibitor hemophilia patients have led to a widening gap in quality of life for inhibitor patients. Further research in hemophilia should have a strong focus on the prevention and treatment of inhibitor patients.

References

1 Darby SC, Keeling DM, Spooner RJ, Wan Kan S, Giangrande PL, Collins PW, Hill FG, Hay CR; UK Haemophilia Centre Doctors' Organisation: The incidence of factor VIII and factor IX inhibitors in the hemophilia population of the UK and their effect on subsequent mortality, 1977–99. J Thromb Haemost 2004;2:1047–1054.

2 Gringeri A, Mantovani LG, Scalone L, Mannucci PM; COCIS Study Group: Cost of care and quality of life for patients with hemophilia complicated by inhibitors: the COCIS study group. Blood 2003;102:2358–2363.

3 Dimichele D: Inhibitors: resolving diagnostic and therapeutic dilemmas. Haemophilia 2002;8:280–287.

4 Barrow RT, Healey JF, Gailani D, Scandella D, Lollar P: Reduction of the antigenicity of factor VIII toward complex inhibitory antibody plasmas using multiply-substituted hybrid human/porcine factor VIII molecules. Blood 2000;95:564–568.

5 Van Der Bom JG, Mauser-Bunschoten EP, Fischer K, Van Den Berg HM: Age at first treatment and immune tolerance to factor VIII in severe hemophilia. Thromb Haemost 2003;89:475–479.

6 Rossi G, Sarkar J, Scandella D: Long-term induction of immune tolerance after blockade of CD40-CD40L interaction in a mouse model of hemophilia A. Blood 2001;97:2750–2757.

7 Qian J, Collins M, Sharpe AH, Hoyer LW: Prevention and treatment of factor VIII inhibitors in murine hemophilia A. Blood 2000;95:1324–1329.

8 Madoiwa S, Yamauchi T, Hakamata Y, Kobayashi E, Arai M, Sugo T, Mimuro J, Sakata Y: Induction of immune tolerance by neonatal intravenous injection of human factor VIII in murine hemophilia A. J Thromb Haemost 2004;2:754–762.

9 Sharathkumar A, Lillicrap D, Blanchette VS, Kern M, Leggo J, Stain AM, Brooker L, Carcao MD: Intensive exposure to factor VIII is a risk factor for inhibitor development in mild hemophilia A. J Thromb Haemost 2003;1:1228–1236.

10 Ewenstein BM, Hoots WK, Lusher JM, Dimichele D, White GC 2nd, Adelman B, Nadeau K: Inhibition of CD40 ligand (CD154) in the treatment of factor VIII inhibitors. Haematologica 2000;85(10 suppl):35–39.

11 Auerswald G, Spranger T, Brackmann HH: The role of plasma-derived factor VIII/von Willebrand factor concentrates in the treatment of hemophilia A patients. Haematologica 2003;88:EREP05.

12 Mathias M, Khair K, Hann I, Liesner R: Rituximab in the treatment of alloimmune factor VIII and IX antibodies in two children with severe haemophilia. Br J Haematol 2004;125:366–368.

13 Villard S, Lacroix-Desmazes S, Kieber-Emmons T, Piquer D, Grailly S, Benhida A, Kaveri SV, Saint-Remy JM, Granier C: Peptide decoys selected by phage display block in vitro and in vivo activity of a human anti-FVIII inhibitor. Blood 2003;102:949–952.

14 Hilgartner M, Aledort L, Andes A, Gill J: Efficacy and safety of vapor-heated anti-inhibitor coagulant complex in hemophilia patients. FEIBA Study Group. Transfusion 1990;30:626–630.

15 Key NS, Aledort LM, Beardsley D, Cooper HA, Davignon G, Ewenstein BM, Gilchrist GS, Gill JC, Glader B, Hoots WK, Kisker CT, Lusher JM, Rosenfield CG, Shapiro AD, Smith H, Taft E: Home treatment of mild to moderate bleeding episodes using recombinant factor VIIa (Novoseven) in haemophiliacs with inhibitors. Thromb Haemost 1998;80:912–918.

16 Seremetis S: Dose optimization of recombinant factor VIIa in the treatment of acute bleeding in haemophilia-associated inhibitors. Blood Coagul Fibrinolysis 2003;14(suppl 1):S29–S30.

17 Kenet G, Lubetsky A, Luboshitz J, Martinowitz U: A new approach to treatment of bleeding episodes in young hemophilia patients: a single bolus megadose of recombinant activated factor VII (NovoSeven). J Thromb Haemost 2003;1:450–455.

18 Key NS, Christie B, Henderson N, Nelsestuen GL: Possible synergy between recombinant factor VIIa and prothrombin complex concentrate in hemophilia therapy. Thromb Haemost 2002;88:60–65.

19 Schneiderman J, Nugent DJ, Young G: Sequential therapy with activated prothrombin complex concentrate and recombinant factor VIIa in patients with severe haemophilia and inhibitors. Haemophilia 2004;10:347–351.

20 Hilgartner MW, Makipernaa A, Dimichele DM: Long-term FEIBA prophylaxis does not prevent progression of existing joint disease. Haemophilia 2003;9:261–268.

21 Saxon BR, Shanks D, Jory CB, Williams V: Effective prophylaxis with daily recombinant factor VIIa (rFVIIa-Novoseven) in a child with high titre inhibitors and a target joint. Thromb Haemost 2001;86:1126–1127.

22 Young G, McDaniel M, Nugent DJ: Prophylactic recombinant factor VIIa in haemophilia patients with inhibitors. Haemophilia 2005;11:203–207.

23 Persson E, Kjalke M, Olsen OH: Rational design of coagulation factor VIIa variants with substantially increased intrinsic activity. Proc Natl Acad Sci USA 2001;98:13583–13588.

24 Tomokiyo K, Nakatomi Y, Araki T, Teshima K, Nakano H, Nakagaki T, Miyamoto S, Funatsu A, Iwanaga S: A novel therapeutic approach combining human plasma-derived factors VIIa and X for haemophiliacs with inhibitors: evidence of a higher thrombin generation rate in vitro and more sustained haemostatic activity in vivo than obtained with factor VIIa alone. Vox Sang 2003;85:290–299.

25 Parker ET, Craddock HN, Barrow RT, Lollar P: Comparative immunogenicity of recombinant B domain-deleted porcine factor VIII and Hyate:C in hemophilia A mice presensitized to human factor VIII. J Thromb Haemost 2004;2:605–611.

26 Bragadottir G, Onundarson PT: Factor-sparing use of the COX-2 inhibitor rofecoxib in haemophilic arthropathy. Haemophilia 2002;8:832–833.

27 Rattray BN, Nugent DJ, Young G: Rofecoxib as adjunctive therapy for haemophilic arthropathy. Haemophilia 2005;11:240–244.
28 Sramek A, Kriek M, Rosendaal FR: Decreased mortality of ischaemic heart disease among carriers of haemophilia. Lancet 2003;362: 351–354.
29 Rosendaal FR, Varekamp I, Smit C, Brocker-Vriends AH, Van Dijck H, Vandenbroucke JP, Hermans J, Suurmeijer TP, Briet E: Mortality and causes of death in Dutch haemophiliacs, 1973–86. Br J Haematol 1989;71:71–76.
30 Graham DJ: Risk of acute cardiac events among patients treated with cyclooxygenase-2 selective and non-selective nonsteroidal anti-inflammatory drugs (abstract 571). 20th Annual Meeting of the International Society for Pharmacoepidemiology Conference on Pharmacoepidemiology, Bordeaux, 2004.
31 White WB, Faich G, Borer JS, Makuch RW: Cardiovascular thrombotic events in arthritis trials of the cyclooxygenase-2 inhibitor celecoxib. Am J Cardiol 2003;92:411–418.
32 Siegel HJ, Luck JV Jr, Siegel ME, Quinones C: Phosphate-32 colloid radiosynovectomy in hemophilia: outcome of 125 procedures. Clin Orthop 2001;392:409–417.
33 Srivastava A: Dose and response in haemophilia – optimization of factor replacement. Br J Haematol 2004;127:12–25.
34 Key NS, Nelsestuen GL: Views on methods for monitoring recombinant factor VIIa in inhibitor patients. Semin Hematol 2004;41(suppl 1):51–54.
35 Ingerslev J, Christiansen K, Calatzis A, Holm M, Sabroe Ebbesen L: Management and monitoring of recombinant activated factor VII. Blood Coagul Fibrinolysis 2000;11(suppl 1): S25–S30.
36 Nugent DJ, Lovejoy A, Nakagawa P, Young G: Successful use of thromboelastography to determine dosing frequency of rFVIIa and FXIII. Blood 2003;102(suppl 1):307a.

Acta Haematologica

Acta Haematol 2006;115:180–185
DOI: 10.1159/000090932

Arterial Ischemic Stroke and Cerebral Venous Thrombosis in Children: A 12-Year Argentinean Registry

Mariana Bonduel[a] Gabriela Sciuccati[a] Mirta Hepner[a] Graciela Pieroni[a] Aurora Feliú Torres[a] Juan Pablo Frontroth[a] Silvia Tenembaum[b]

[a]Servicio de Hematología-Oncología and [b]Servicio de Neurología, Hospital de Pediatría 'Prof. Dr. Juan P. Garrahan', Buenos Aires, Argentina

Key Words
Acenocoumarol · Children · Stroke · Thrombophilia

Abstract
Over a 12-year period, 112 consecutive children with arterial ischemic stroke (AIS) and 38 children with cerebral venous thrombosis (CVT) were prospectively recruited at a single pediatric center in Argentina. One or more underlying clinical conditions were identified in most patients (55%) with AIS and in almost all patients with CVT. Inherited and/or acquired prothrombotic disorders were detected in 17% of the patients with AIS and in 34% of the children with CVT. No associations between factor V Leiden or prothrombin G20210A mutation and children with AIS or CVT were found. Antithrombotic agents (i.e., aspirin, low-molecular-weight heparin and acenocoumarol) were administered without major hemorrhagic complications. In our cohorts, mortality due to the thrombotic episode was 1.8% in children with AIS. No child with CVT died from his or her thrombotic episodes. Three children (3.2%) and 1 adolescent (1.1%) with AIS had thrombotic progression and recurrence, respectively. A large percentage of children with AIS (68%) and CVT (32%) have had some kind of sequels that caused serious disability in approximately half the cases.

Introduction

Over the last decade, arterial ischemic stroke (AIS) and cerebral venous thrombosis (CVT) have been increasingly recognized as different entities associated with high morbidity and potential mortality [1]. However, several years ago, an estimated incidence of pediatric AIS of 1.2 cases/100,000 children/year was reported in the United States [2] and recent studies from Canada [3] and Germany [4] described estimated incidences of CVT of 0.67 and 0.35/100,000 children/year, respectively; it is now thought that these entities have probably been underdiagnosed [1].

Until now, a few prospective studies with relatively large pediatric series from Argentina [5, 6], Canada [3, 7], Germany [4, 8], UK [9, 10] and Israel [11, 12] have focused on different aspects of AIS and CVT in children.

In 1992 a prospective registry of AIS and CVT was established in the largest pediatric center in Argentina, a developing country with a distinctive ethnic background and geographical distribution. The aim of this study is to report the prospectively collected data over a 12-year period including baseline demographics, clinical data, radiological and laboratory findings in one of the largest pediatric cohort. Within a median follow-up time of 4.4 years (3 months to 11.8 years), the antithrombotic drugs used and outcomes are also described.

KARGER

Fax +41 61 306 12 34
E-Mail karger@karger.ch
www.karger.com

0001–5792/06/1154–0180$23.50/0

Accessible online at:
www.karger.com/aha

Mariana Bonduel, MD
Servicio de Hematología-Oncología, Hospital de Pediatría 'Prof. Dr. Juan P. Garrahan'
Combate de los Pozos 1881, C1245AAM Buenos Aires (Argentina)
Tel. +54 11 4308 0927, Fax +54 11 4308 5325
E-Mail mbonduel@garrahan.gov.ar or mbonduel@yahoo.com

Patients and Methods

In May 1992, a registry of AIS and CVT was initiated at the Haematology Department of the Hospital de Pediatría 'Prof. Dr. Juan P. Garrahan', Buenos Aires, Argentina. This is the largest tertiary pediatric center in Argentina where children coming from all over the country are treated. The inclusion criteria encompassed infants and children aged from 0.2 months to 18 years with first onset of the thrombotic episode. Newborns and patients with moyamoya syndrome were excluded from this study for additional evaluation. The thrombotic events were confirmed by computed tomography, magnetic resonance imaging, magnetic resonance angiography and/or arteriography.

From May 1992 to November 2004, 112 consecutive patients with AIS and 38 patients with CVT were enrolled in this registry. Each patient was evaluated by the hematologists involved in this study and a neurologist at the beginning and at a minimum of once yearly. A standardized history including clinical presentation, personal and family history of thrombosis, underlying disorders and/or circumstantial risk factors, radiological studies, laboratory findings, treatment and outcomes was updated at each visit. All data were collected prospectively.

The laboratory evaluation began after having obtained informed parental consent. Blood samples were collected into 0.11 *M* sodium citrate at a ratio of 9:1 by clean venipuncture. Blood was centrifuged at 2,500 *g* for 10 min to obtain platelet-poor plasma. The platelet-poor plasma was then centrifuged for a further 5 min at 2,500 *g* and plasma was immediately processed or stored in 1-ml aliquots at –70°C. For DNA analysis blood was collected into glass vacutainer tubes containing EDTA (Becton Dickinson Vacutainer® Systems, Franklin Lakes, N.J., USA). DNA was extracted from white cell fraction using DNAzol® reagent (Life Technologies, Grand Island, N.Y., USA).

To determine factor V Leiden (FVL) and prothrombin G20210A mutation (PT20210A) simultaneously, we performed a multiplex allele-specific amplification PCR as previously described in patients and controls [13]. Nine children, who were admitted between 1992 and 1994, were recalled later in order to obtain DNA samples. DNA samples were available from 98 of 112 (88%) children with AIS and from all patients with CVT.

Evaluation for prothrombotic disorders included the following assays: prothrombin time, activated partial thromboplastin time, thrombin time, reptilase time, fibrinogen and factor V activity by standard procedures. Functional activities of protein C (PC), antithrombin (AT) and plasminogen (PLG) were measured by amidolytic assays (Chromogenix, Mölndal, Sweden) and PC and protein S (PS) by clotting assays (Diagnostica Stago, Asnières, France) using a model ST4 coagulometer (Diagnostica Stago). PC antigen was measured by a commercial ELISA kit (Diagnostica Stago). Immunologic measurements of PS (total and free), AT and PLG were made by Laurell's technique using polyclonal rabbit antibodies against the respective antigens (PS, and AT, Dakopatts, Denmark; Assera PLG, Diagnostica Stago) [14]. Free PS was assayed by precipitating bound protein with polyethylene glycol 8000 (3.75%) according to the method by Comp et al. [15]. The presence of activated PC resistance was tested using a commercial kit with factor V-deficient plasma as a prediluent for plasma samples (Chromogenix AB; Mölndal, Sweden). The presence of a lupus anticoagulant (LA) was determined based on abnormal screening assays, mixing studies and confirmatory assays based on the method giving abnormal screening test results [16]. The tests used were activated partial thromboplastin time (PTT-LA, Diagnostica Stago) and diluted Russell viper venom time (Sigma-Aldrich, St. Louis, Mo., USA) with confirmation using the platelet neutralization procedure as recommended by the International Society on Thrombosis and Haemostasis [17]. Sera for anticardiolipin antibodies (ACA) were assayed for IgG and IgM isotypes using an in-house ELISA previously described [18], calibrated against Dr. Harris' standards from the University of Louisville, Kentucky. According to proposed criteria for the antiphospholipid syndrome (APS), only those patients with positive LA test results and/or positive IgG and/or IgM ACA at moderate/high levels (>20 GPL or MPL units) in two determinations performed more than 6 weeks apart were considered positive for APS [19]. LA and ACA were tested within 1 month after the thrombotic event in all cases. Their parents were also studied to exclude familial APS.

A thrombophilia study was carried out in all the patients recruited in the registry. In children with cerebral thrombosis and ALL, the assay for the detection of acquired AT deficiency was performed immediately after the thrombotic episode was radiologically confirmed.

At least 3–6 months after the thrombotic event, the evaluation for inherited prothrombotic disorders was carried out. The final diagnosis was made when repeatedly measured plasma concentrations of the coagulation proteins investigated were outside the age-appropriate reference ranges. The finding of the same abnormal laboratory results in the parents confirmed the suspected inherited coagulation defect.

In children who were under oral anticoagulation, plasma samples were obtained 15–30 days after withdrawal of the therapy.

With informed parental consent, a total of 102 healthy children (60 males/42 females, median age 7.1 years, range 0.2–15.9 years) admitted to the hospital for elective minor surgery or as potential bone marrow donors were eligible for reference ranges and as a control group for DNA analysis.

Statistical Analysis

For comparison, Fisher's exact test was used. Odds ratios and 95% confidence intervals were calculated for FVL and PT20210A. Statistical significance was taken as a p value ≤ 0.05 for two extremes. The software used was CSS/Statistica, 5.1 (StatSoft, Tulsa, Okla., USA) [20, 21].

Results

Over a 12-year period, 112 consecutive children with AIS and 38 children with CVT were enrolled in this registry. Twenty-one children with the moyamoya syndrome were excluded from further analysis. Data of baseline demographics, clinical data, underlying diseases and/or circumstantial risk factors, symptoms and signs, radiological findings and family history of thrombosis of these cohorts are shown in table 1.

In children with AIS, the median age at the first thrombotic episode was 5.5 years (range 0.2–17.1 years). The youngest patients of this cohort (median age 1.6 years,

Table 1. Patients' characteristics

	AIS (n = 112)	CVT (n = 38)
Age		
>2 months to <1 year	17	6
≥1 to <6 years	42	9
≥6 to <11 years	24	14
≥11 to ≤18 years	29	9
Age median (range), years	5.5 (0.2–17.1)	7.7 (0.2–15.4)
F/M	49/63	11/27
Underlying disease and/or circumstantial risk factor		
Cardiac diseases	27	–
Infection	24	19
Head trauma	7	2
ALL with ASP therapy	3	6
Non-Hodgkin's lymphoma	1	2
Dehydration	–	2
ALL	1	2
Systemic lupus erythematosus	2	1
Hodgkin's disease	–	1
Biliary atresia	1	–
Non-Hodgkin's lymphoma with ASP therapy	–	1
Tumors of the central nervous system	–	2
Hyperlipidemia type IV	1	–
None	50	3
Symptoms and signs		
Hemiparesis	70	11
Headache	35	36
Seizures	37	18
Change in mental status	18	21
Aphasia	14	–
Ataxia	12	–
Others	3	–
Radiological findings		
Left middle cerebral artery occlusion	41	–
Right middle cerebral artery occlusion	38	–
Posterior cerebral artery occlusion	12	–
Multiple arterial thrombosis	9	–
Carotid artery occlusion	5	–
Vertebral artery occlusion	5	–
Basilar artery occlusion	2	–
Superior sagittal sinovenous thrombosis	–	18
Lateral sinovenous thrombosis	–	7
Sagittal and straight sinovenous thrombosis	–	5
Sagittal and lateral sinovenous thrombosis	–	5
Sagittal and internal cerebral vein thrombosis	–	3
Family history of thrombosis	7	5

ALL = Acute lymphoblastic leukemia; ASP = *L*-asparaginase.

range 0.2–15 years) were those with previously recognized cardiac diseases. There was a male predominance (ratio of males to females was 1.3 to 1). Underlying clinical conditions and/or circumstantial risk factors were detected in 62 patients (55%). The most frequent clinical factors reported were cardiac diseases (24%) and infectious diseases (21%). Only 1 patient had chickenpox within the previous year. Although transthoracic echocardiography was conducted soon after the thrombotic episode in all patients, intracardiac thrombosis was not identified in any case. A positive family history of thrombosis was found in 7 patients (6%). In most patients (71%) with AIS,

Table 2. Laboratory findings

	AIS (n = 112)	CVT (n = 38)
Inherited prothrombotic disorders		
AT deficiency	–	1
PC deficiency	1	–
PS deficiency	2	–
FVL	2	1
PT20210A	1	1
Combined prothrombotic disorders		
FVL/inherited PC deficiency	–	1
PT20210A/inherited PC deficiency	–	1
Inherited plasminogen deficiency/LA	1	–
Acquired prothrombotic disorders		
AT deficiency	4	6
LA	3	2
ACA	4	–
LA and ACA	1	–
Total	19 (17%)	13 (34%)

PT20210A = Prothrombin G20210A mutation.

brain lesions were found in the territories of the middle cerebral arteries (left middle cerebral arteries; 52%). Inherited and/or acquired prothrombotic disorders were found in 19 patients (17%) (data summarized in table 2). The frequencies of FVL of patients and controls were 1.8 and 2.0%, respectively (OR = 1.1, CI 95%: 0.15–7.96, p = 1). The frequencies of PT20210A of patients and controls were 0.9 and 1.0%, respectively (OR = 1.1, CI 95%: 0.07–17.8, p = 1). Antithrombotic therapy was given to all patients. Since the diagnosis was confirmed, 84 patients (75%) have been receiving aspirin 5 mg/kg/day and 27 children (24%; 24 patients had congenital heart diseases, 2 patients had cardiomyopathy and the remaining child had a persistent LA) have been under acenocoumarol therapy to maintain an INR of 2.0–2.5. No major hemorrhagic complications were observed. No patient receiving acenocoumarol therapy presented a recurrent thrombotic episode. Six patients died during the acute episode, 2 of them (1.8%) from the thrombotic event and the remaining 4 from their underlying diseases. Fourteen patients were lost to follow-up. Ninety-two children were followed up for a median of 4.8 years (5 months to 11.8 years). Three children (3.2%) and 1 adolescent (1.1%) had thrombotic progression and recurrence, respectively. After the recurrence these children were placed on acenocoumarol therapy and no new thrombotic episode has been observed. Sixty-three children (68%) showed different kinds of neurological sequels (data shown in table 3).

Table 3. Patients' outcomes

	AIS	CVT
Mortality		
Recruited patients	112	38
Due to underlying clinical condition	4	7
Due to thrombosis	2	–
Morbidity		
Evaluable patients[1]	92	31
Thrombotic progression	3	–
Thrombotic recurrence	1	–
Neurological sequels	63 (68%)	10 (32%)
Hemiplegia	35	4
Cognitive impairment	13	3
Mild motor deficit	11	–
Convulsive disorder	5	2
Aphasia	4	–
Severe visual impairment	2	–
Ataxia	1	–
Pseudotumor cerebri	–	2

[1] Lost to follow-up: 14 AIS patients (12.5%) and 1 CVT patient (3%).

In children with CVT, the median age at the first thrombotic episode was 7.7 years. There was a male predominance (ratio of males to females was 2.5 to 1). At least one underlying clinical condition was present in 35 patients (92%). In 5 patients (13%) a positive family history of thrombosis was found. Thirty-one patients (82%) had thrombosis of the superior sagittal sinus. Inherited and/or acquired prothrombotic disorders were identified in 13 patients (34%; data summarized in table 2). The frequencies of FVL from patients and controls were 5.3 and 2.0%, respectively (OR = 0.36, CI 95%: 0.05–2.65, p = 0.5744). The frequencies of PT20210A from patients and controls were 5.3 and 1.0%, respectively (OR = 0.8, CI 95%: 0.02–2.03, p = 0.1791). As initial therapy, 26 patients (68%) without intracranial hemorrhage and no high risk of bleeding received the low-molecular-weight heparin (LMWH) enoxaparin for 2 weeks. All patients were under oral anticoagulation therapy for 3 months to maintain an INR between 2.0 and 3.0. No major hemorrhagic complications were observed. Seven patients died from their underlying diseases during the acute episode. No patient died from thrombotic complications. One child was lost to follow-up. Thirty children were followed up for a median of 3.8 years (3 months to 11.5 years), no patient developed recurrent thrombosis upon cessation of oral anticoagulation therapy and 10 patients (32%) had different kinds of sequels.

Discussion

Over the last decade, AIS and CVT have been increasingly recognized as underdiagnosed pediatric disorders that underlie mortality and considerable morbidity [1]. Multiple underlying clinical conditions have been recognized in pediatric AIS and CVT [1–5, 8, 10, 12]. The recognition of several patients subtypes has hindered making the most appropriate radiological and laboratory diagnosis, and the prevention and treatment of these entities. In our registry, one or more underlying clinical conditions were identified in most children with AIS and in almost all patients with CVT. Our hospital treats a large population of children with acute lymphoblastic leukemia who receive *L*-asparaginase as part of their treatment [20]. A more thorough radiological and laboratory testing performed in the large number of children (45%) with idiopathic AIS could have identified uncommon risk factors (i.e., vasculopathies, metabolic disorders, mitochondrial diseases). The association of prothrombotic disorders with childhood AIS or CVT is still controversial. The published frequencies of these prothrombotic disorders vary widely in the literature [4–9, 11, 12, 22–24]. The combination of lipoprotein (a) and PC deficiency with an underlying condition was reported as independent associations with CVT in German children [4]. A study from Israel found that thrombophilia was more frequent among children with idiopathic CVT [12]. As is the case in other publications [9, 23–25], in the current study a lower frequency of inherited and/or acquired prothrombotic disorders was detected when compared to data reported by some other pediatric series [7, 8, 11, 26], and no association between FVL or prothrombin G20210A mutation and children with AIS or CVT was found in these cohorts. This fact may be partially explained by different sample sizes, inclusion criteria, control group selection, as well as distinctive ethnic background and geographical distribution. The proposal of antithrombotic therapy remains a matter of discussion until evidence-based data on efficacy and safety are determined [27].

A low dose of aspirin was used as a lifelong therapy in all children with AIS in our cohort. Meanwhile, the patients with cardiac diseases as a probable embolic source, such as arterial dissection, persistence of an APS or thrombotic recurrence, were placed on acenocoumarol therapy until the predisposing risk factor was no longer present. Acenocoumarol therapy was used considering different loading doses according to age [28]. In children with CVT, without intracranial hemorrhage and no high risk of bleeding, LMWH was used during 2 weeks soon after the thrombosis was radiologically confirmed. After this initial therapy, acenocoumarol therapy was administered during 3 months or until the predisposing risk factor was no longer present. No child had major hemorrhagic complications.

In our cohorts, mortality due to the thrombotic episode was 1.8% in children with AIS. No child with CVT died from the thrombotic episode. A large percentage of children with AIS (68%) and CVT (32%) have had some kind of sequels that caused serious disability in approximately half the cases. A multicenter international prospective study with a large cohort of pediatric patients from a similar ethnic background is needed to establish which combinations of prothrombotic disorders with underlying clinical conditions are associated with the different patient subtypes of AIS and CVT, and also to determine the optimal antithrombotic therapies.

References

1 Andrew M, Monagle PT, Brooker L: Stroke; in Andrew M, Monagle PT, Brooker L (eds): Thromboembolic Complications during Infancy and Childhood. London, Decker, 2000, pp 47–110.

2 Schoenberg BS, Mellinger JF, Schoenberg DF: Cerebrovascular disease in infants and children: a study of incidence, clinical features, and survival. Neurology 1978;28:763–768.

3 deVeber G, Andrew M, Adams C, Bjornson B, Booth F, Buckley DJ, Camfield CS, David M, Humphreys P, Langevin P, MacDonald EA, Meaney B, Shevell M, Sinclair DB, Yager J, Gillett J: Cerebral sinovenous thrombosis in children. N Engl J Med 2001;345:417–423.

4 Heller C, Heinecke A, Junker R, Knöfler R, Kosch A, Kurnik K, Schobess R, von Eckardstein A, Sträter R, Zieger B, Nowak-Göttl U; Childhood Stroke Study Group: Cerebral venous thrombosis in children. A multifactorial origin. Circulation 2003;108:1362–1367.

5 Bonduel M, Sciuccati G, Hepner M, Torres AF, Pieroni G, Frontroth JP: Prethrombotic disorders in children with arterial ischemic stroke and sinovenous thrombosis. Arch Neurol 1999;56:967–971.

6 Bonduel M, Sciuccati G, Hepner M, Pieroni G, Torres AF, Mardaraz C, Frontroth JP: Factor V Leiden and prothrombin gene G20210A mutation in children with cerebral thromboembolism. Am J Hematol 2003;73:81–86.

7 deVeber G, Monagle P, Chan A, MacGregor D, Curtis R, Lee S, Vegh P, Adams M, Marzinotto V, Leaker M, Massicotte P, Lillicrap D, Andrew M: Prothrombotic disorders in infants and children with cerebral thromboembolism. Arch Neurol 1998;55:1539–1543.

8 Nowak-Göttl U, Sträter R, Heinecke A, Junker R, Koch HG, Schuierer G, von Eckardstein A: Lipoprotein (a) and genetic polymorphisms of clotting factor V, prothrombin and methylenetetrahydrofolate reductase are risk factors of spontaneous ischemic stroke in children. Blood 1999;94:3678–3682.

9 Ganesan V, McShane MA, Liesner R, Cookson J, Hann I, Kirkham FJ: Inherited prothrombotic states and ischaemic stroke in childhood. J Neurol Neurosurg Psychiatry 1998;65:508–511.

10 Ganesan V, Prengler M, McShane MA, Wade AM, Kirkham FJ: Investigation of risk factors in children with arterial ischemic stroke. Ann Neurol 2003;53:167–173.

11 Kenet G, Sadetzki S, Murad H, Martinowitz U, Rosenberg N, Gitel S, Rechavi G, Inbal A: Factor V Leiden and antiphospholipid antibodies are significant risk factors for ischemic stroke in children. Stroke 2000;31:1283–1288.

12 Kenet G, Waldman D, Lubetsky A, Kornbrut N, Khalil A, Koren A, Wolach B, Fattal A, Kapelushnik J, Tamary H, Yacobovitch J, Raveh E, Revel-Vilk S, Toren A, Brenner B: Paediatric cerebral sinus vein thrombosis. A multi-center, case-controlled study. Thromb Haemost 2004;92:713–718.

13 Hézard N, Cornillet-Lefebvre P, Gillot L, Potron L, Nguyen P: Multiplex ASA PCR for a simultaneous determination of factor V Leiden gene, G→A 20210 prothrombin gene and C→T 677 MTHFR gene mutations. Thromb Haemost 1998;79:1054–1055.

14 Laurell CB: Electroimmuno assay Scand J Clin Lab Invest 1972;29:21–37.

15 Comp PC, Nixon RR, Cooper MR, Esmon CT: Familial protein S deficiency is associated with thrombosis. J Clin Invest 1984;74:2082–2088.

16 Brandt JT, Triplett DA, Alvin B, Scharrer I: Criteria for the diagnosis of lupus anticoagulants: an update. On behalf of the Subcommittee on Lupus Anticoagulant/Antiphospholipid Antibody of the Scientific and Standardization Committee of the ISTH. Thromb Haemost 1995;74:1185–1190.

17 Triplett DA, Brandt JT, Kaczor D, Schaeffer J: Laboratory diagnosis of lupus inhibitors: a comparison of the tissue thromboplastin inhibition procedure with a new platelet neutralization procedure. Am J Clin Pathol 1983;79:678–682.

18 Harris EN, Gharavi AE, Patel SP, Hughes GR: Evaluation of the anticardiolipin antibody test: report of an international workshop held 4 April 1986. Clin Exp Immunol 1987;68:215–222.

19 Harris EN, Khamashta MA, Hughes GRV: Antiphospholipid antibody syndrome; in Mc Carthy DJ, Koopman WJ (eds): Arthritis and Allied Conditions, ed 12. Philadelphia, Lea & Febiger, 1991, pp 1201–1212.

20 Amitage P, Berry G: Statistical methods in medical research; in Further Analysis of Categorical Data. Oxford, Blackwell, 1994.

21 Rothman K, Greenland S: Case control studies; in Rothman K, Greenland S (eds): Modern Epidemiology, ed 2. Philadelphia, Lippincott-Raven, 1998, pp 93–114.

22 Bonduel M, Sciuccati G, Hepner M, Feliú Torres A, Sackmann Muriel F: Thrombosis in children with acute lymphoblastic leukaemia (ALL) and *L*-asparaginase (ASP) therapy (abstract). Blood 1997;90:3756.

23 McColl MD, Chalmers EA, Thomas A, Sproul A, Healey C, Rafferty I, McWilliam R, Eunson P: Factor V Leiden, prothrombin 20210G→A and the MTHFR C677T mutations in childhood stroke. Thromb Haemost 1999;81:690–694.

24 Riikonen RS, Santavuori P: Hereditary and acquired risk factors for childhood stroke. Neuropediatrics 1994;25:227.

25 Riikonen RS, Vahtera EM, Kekomäki RM: Physiological anticoagulants and activated protein C resistance in childhood stroke. Acta Paediatr 1996;85:242–244.

26 Becker S, Heller C, Gropp F, Scharrer I, Kreuz W: Thrombophilic disorders in children with cerebral infarction. Lancet 1998;352:1756–1757.

27 Monagle P, Chan A, Massicotte P, Chalmers E, Michelson AD: Antithrombotic therapy in children: the Seventh ACCP Conference on Antithrombotic and Thrombolytic Therapy. Chest 2004;126:645S–687S.

28 Bonduel M, Sciuccati G, Hepner M, Torres AF, Pieroni G, Frontroth JP, Serviddio RM: Acenocoumarol therapy in pediatric patients. J Thromb Haemost 2003;1:740–743.

Acta Haematologica

Acta Haematol 2006;115:186–191
DOI: 10.1159/000090933

Elevated α_1-Antitrypsin Is a Risk Factor for Arterial Ischemic Stroke in Childhood

Beate Burghaus[a] Claus Langer[b, c] Sabine Thedieck[a] Ulrike Nowak-Göttl[a]

[a]Department of Paediatric Haematology and Oncology, [b]Institute of Clinical Chemistry and [c]Institute of Arteriosclerosis Research, University of Münster, Münster, Germany

Key Words

α_1-Antitrypsin · Factor V G1691A · Lipoprotein (a) · Thromboembolism, pediatric

Abstract

α_1-antitrypsin (α_1-AT) is a physiological inhibitor of activated protein C (APC) and therefore decreased APC activity. APC itself causes an anticoagulant effect by inactivating factors Va and VIIIa. The present case-control study was performed to evaluate the role of the elevated α_1-AT concentration in pediatric patients with ischemic stroke (IS). α_1-AT concentrations were measured along with established prothrombotic risk factors 6–12 months after the acute thrombotic onset in 81 Caucasian children with IS aged 1 month to 18 years. The cutoff values defined as age-dependent 90th percentiles were obtained from 229 healthy controls. Median (range) values of α_1-AT were significantly higher in patients compared with control subjects [122.0 mg/dl (61.4–224.0) vs. 114.0 mg/dl (66.8–156.0); p = 0.016]. In addition, 14 of the 81 patients (17.3%) compared with 10 of the 162 controls (6.2%) had α_1-AT concentrations above the 90th age-dependent percentiles (p = 0.012). Multivariate analysis performed in a 1:2 matched case-control setting adjusted for the presence of established prothrombotic risk factors showed a significantly increased odds ratio (OR) and 95% confidence interval (CI) for patients with elevated α_1-AT >90th percentiles and IS (OR/CI: 4.0/1.64–9.92; p = 0.0024). Data shown here give evidence that total α_1-AT concentrations above the 90th age-dependent percentiles independently increase the risk of IS 4.0-fold in Caucasian children.

Introduction

Although venous and arterial thromboses are rare diseases in infancy and childhood, incidences of symptomatic thrombotic manifestations are recorded in 0.07/10,000 children, in 5.3/10,000 admissions of children and 2.4/1,000 admissions of newborns to intensive care units [1, 2]. It has been reported that several clinical and environmental conditions, such as peripartal asphyxia, neonatal infections, fetal diabetes, the use of central lines, trauma or surgery, dehydration, malignant disease, renal disease, autoimmune disease, or the application of oral contraceptives by adolescent girls resulted in elevated thrombin generation with subsequent thrombus formation in infancy and childhood, e.g. venous thrombosis or ischemic stroke (IS) of thromboembolic origin [1, 3–7]. However, before the era of extensive molecular testing in many children the etiopathology of thromboembolic events remained unclear.

KARGER

Fax +41 61 306 12 34
E-Mail karger@karger.ch
www.karger.com

0001–5792/06/1154–0186$23.50/0

Accessible online at:
www.karger.com/aha

U. Nowak-Göttl
Paediatric Haematology and Oncology, University Children's Hospital
Albert-Schweitzer-Strasse 33
DE–48149 Münster (Germany)
Tel. +49 251 834 7936/7744, Fax +49 251 834 7828, E-Mail leagottl@uni-muenster.de

Various genetic defects of proteins regulating blood coagulation have been established as risk factors for thromboembolic diseases. Most of them affect the protein C pathway, namely activated protein C (APC) resistance, in the majority of cases due to the factor V mutation, as well as deficiencies of protein C and protein S due to other causes. Prothrombotic states have also been associated with defects in the genes of antithrombin, plasminogen, and fibrinogen [8–10]. In addition, the previously described G20210A variant of the factor II gene also seems to be a common but probably mild risk factor for arterial and venous thromboembolism [11, 12]. Furthermore, prothrombotic states are associated with metabolic diseases such as increased fasting total homocysteine plasma levels [13] as well as elevated concentrations of lipoprotein (a) [Lp(a)] [14]. As recently shown, 40–50% of symptomatic thromboembolism in pediatric Caucasian cohorts are attributable to genetic prothrombotic risk factors.

With the intention to further close the gap between the unclear cases of pediatric stroke with respect to prothrombotic risk factors associated with defects within the protein C pathway, in the present evaluation we focused on a physiological plasma protein that has been described as an inhibitor of APC, namely α_1-antitrypsin (α_1-AT) [15, 16]. Inhibiting APC, elevated α_1-AT could theoretically mimic a 'protein C-deficient state' subsequently leading to a prothrombotic situation. To investigate the role of elevated α_1-AT as a candidate risk factor for symptomatic IS in children the present case-control study was performed.

Material and Methods

Ethics

The present study was performed in accordance with the ethical standards laid down in the updated relevant version of Declaration of Helsinki and approved by the medical ethics committee at the Westfälische Wilhelms University, Münster, Germany.

Patients

Caucasian pediatric patients with a first symptomatic thromboembolic event were consecutively recruited and screened for hereditary prothrombotic risk factors between January 1996 and June 2003 by the participating centers in the catchment areas of Hamburg, Kiel, Lübeck, Münster, Bielefeld, Düsseldorf, Berlin, Magdeburg, Halle, and Munich.

Inclusion Criteria

Neonates, infants and children aged 1 month to 18 years with the first onset of a thromboembolic stroke event were included. A thromboembolic stroke event had to be confirmed objectively by standard imaging methods, i.e. cerebral CT scanning, MR imaging, MR angiography, or transcranial Doppler ultrasonography.

Exclusion Criteria

Patients older than 18 years, children not of Caucasian origin, patients with incomplete clinical or laboratory workup (established prothrombotic risk factors), and children lost to follow-up or without parental consent were not enrolled in the present study. In addition, children during the acute thromboembolic phase, patients with renal insufficiency, liver disease or malignancies, and adolescent girls taking oral contraceptives were excluded.

Final Study Population

From the ongoing multicenter study a randomly selected subgroup of 81 pediatric patients with a median age of 2.5 years (range: 1 month to 18 years) was enrolled. Randomization into the substudy – and therefore reduction of the patient number – was performed to achieve standard conditions. For the case-control design a 1:2 matching was performed.

Control Group

A total of 229 healthy children were investigated to determine the age-dependent levels of α_1-AT and the age-dependent percentiles. Controls were recruited between January 1996 and June 2003. Control children had no history of chronic disease or thromboembolic events and were medication-free at the time of enrolment. They presented as outpatients for evaluation before minor surgery or were potential bone marrow donors.

Laboratory Tests

With informed parental consent, the factor V G1691A (FV) and factor II G20210A (FII) mutations, concentration of Lp(a), protein C, protein S, antithrombin, total fasting plasma homocysteine levels and total α_1-AT levels were investigated in patients and controls 6–12 months after the acute event, using standard laboratory techniques [12–17]. In patients and controls peripheral venipuncture was performed in the morning between 8 and 10 a.m. after a standardized fasting period: at least 4 h for infants below 1 year of age including breast-fed infants, and more than 8 h for children above 1 year of age. Blood samples were collected by peripheral venipuncture into plastic tubes containing 1/10 by volume of 3.8% trisodium citrate (Sarstedt, Nümbrecht, Germany), and placed immediately on melting ice. Platelet-poor plasma was prepared by centrifugation at 2,000 *g* for 15 min at 4°C 2 times, aliquoted in polystyrene tubes, stored at –70°C, and thawed immediately before the assay procedure. Total α_1-AT was investigated with a commercially available antiserum against α_1-AT (Dade Behring, Marburg, Germany) in a Behring Nephelometer II, BN II (Dade Behring).

Statistical Analysis

All statistical analyses were performed with the StatView 5 software package (SAS Institute) and the MedCalc software package (MedCalc, Mariakerke, Belgium). Prevalence rates of prothrombotic risk factors in patients and control subjects were calculated by χ^2 analysis or by Fisher's exact test. To compare the overall rate of prothrombotic risk factors between patients and controls and to evaluate the interaction between elevated α_1-AT concentrations and established prothrombotic risk factors, odds ratios (ORs) together with 95% confidence intervals (CIs) were estimated from a multivariate analysis using a logistic regression model. The significance level was set at 0.05. For variables with a non-Gaussian frequency distribution data were presented as median and ranges. The Mann-Whitney test was used to compare median (range) values obtained in patients and controls, and Spearman's rank test was used to calculate correlations between total α_1-AT levels and age. p values <0.05 were considered significant.

Results

Distribution of α_1-AT Levels in Healthy Children

The total median concentration of α_1-AT was 114.0 mg/dl (range: 66.8–207.0) in 229 control subjects tested. In addition, in accordance with literature reports and similar to other components of the hemostatic system during childhood [18–20], age dependency was shown (p = 0.045; rho = 0.16). In table 1 age-dependent median (range) levels of α_1-AT concentrations are demonstrated. Infants from 1 to 12 months had a median α_1-AT concentration of 103.5 mg/dl and children from 1.1 to 4.0 years had a median α_1-AT concentration of 112.0 mg/dl, with a further α_1-AT increase noted in older children from 4.1 to 9.0 and up to 18 years (115.0 mg/dl).

Cutoffs Used for Case-Control Study

Similar to median (range) α_1-AT concentrations the upper 90th age-dependent percentiles were determined within the healthy pediatric population. In the youngest age group (1–12 months) the upper 90th percentile was 130.3 mg/dl. Children between 1.1 and 4.0 years showed a cutoff of 144.2 mg/dl, and in subjects between 4.1 and 9.0 years the upper 90th percentile of α_1-AT was 147.2 mg/dl. During late childhood and puberty (9.1–18.0 years) the cutoff for α_1-AT levels decreased towards adult values (140.0 mg/dl).

α_1-AT Concentrations in Patients and Controls

In patients with IS (n = 81) the median level of α_1-AT was 122.0 mg/dl (range 61.4–224.0 mg/dl), whereas in control children (n = 162) the median concentration was significantly lower (114.0 mg/dl, range 66.8–156.0 mg/dl; p = 0.016). In the group of children with stroke, 14 of 81 patients (17.3%) versus 10 of the 162 children (6.2%) in the control group had α_1-AT levels above the age-specific 90th percentile (p = 0.012).

Multivariate Analysis

Logistic regression was performed in a 1:2 matched design (81 patients compared with 162 controls). Table 2 shows the interaction between elevated α_1-AT and established prothrombotic risk factors. Including the overall

Table 1. Concentrations of α_1-AT and upper 90th percentiles in a cohort of healthy Caucasian children

Age years	α_1-AT levels mg/dl	90th percentiles mg/dl
0.1–1.0	103.5 (79.3–135.0) n = 32	130.3
1.1–4.0	112.0 (69.6–191.0) n = 53	144.2
4.1–9.0	115.0 (66.8–207.0) n = 69	147.2
9.1–18.0	115.0 (76.9–195.0) n = 75	140.0
Total	114.0 (66.8–207.0) n = 229	139.2

α_1-AT levels are given as median with the range in parentheses.

Table 2. Distribution of single and combined prothrombotic risk factors in patients and healthy age-matched controls

Prothrombotic risk factor (total α_1-AT >90th percentiles)	Patients (n = 81)	Controls (n = 162)	p value
Single	14/81 (17.3%)	10/162 (6.2%)	0.01
Combined	48/81 (59.3%)	46/162 (28.4%)	<0.000
With factor V G1691A	16	8	
With factor II G20210A	6	4	
With Lp(a) >30 mg/dl	25	34	
With protein C type I deficiency	1	0	
With protein S type I deficiency	0	0	
With antithrombin type I deficiency	0	0	
Sum of single and combined	62/81 (76.5%)	56/162 (34.6%)	<0.000

rate of established prothrombotic risk factors known to be significantly associated with symptomatic thromboembolism in pediatric patients in Germany, e.g. the FV G1691A mutation, the FII G20210A variant, deficiency states of protein C, S or antithrombin, or elevated Lp(a) concentrations with an overall OR/CI of 2.9/1.6–5.3 ($p = 0.0004$), elevated α_1-AT levels greater than the age-specific 90th percentiles retained their statistically significant and independent association (OR/CI 4.0/1.6–9.9; $p = 0.002$).

Discussion

APC is an anticoagulant serine protease in plasma. It downregulates the coagulation cascade by degrading the procoagulant factors Va and VIIIa by limited proteolysis. Factors Va and VIIIa are obligatory cofactors for thrombin generation. The proteolytic activity of APC in plasma among other factors is regulated by members of the serpin (serine protease inhibitor) family of proteins, e.g. protein C inhibitor, plasminogen activator inhibitor and α_1-AT [15, 16, 21, 22]. α_1-AT inactivates APC by forming a 1:1 stoichiometric complex [16]. By forming this complex a conformational change occurs in α_1-AT, which results in a significant stabilization relative to the noncomplexed serpin α_1-AT [23–25]. The inactivation of APC by α_1-AT is relatively low, and not influenced by heparin [15, 16]. Despite its low interaction with APC, based on its high concentration in plasma, α_1-AT is discussed to be a physiological and important factor for the regulation of APC activity in plasma, especially in the absence of heparin [15, 16, 26, 27]. Furthermore, it has been suggested that α_1-AT becomes the major inhibitor of APC when protein C inhibitor is depleted by an increasing APC generation [28, 29].

Data on the possible association between α_1-AT concentrations and IS are sparse and controversial. Fletcher et al. [30] described that α_1-AT concentrations in adult patients with cerebral infarction were significantly increased in comparison to controls, and Bartosik-Psujek et al. [31] found elevated levels of α_1-AT in adult patients with cerebral ischemia. The latter authors determined α_1-AT in the acute phase of stroke events within the first 7 days and, therefore, interpret their results as indicating that ischemic necrosis is associated with inflammatory reactions. Furthermore, significantly increased α_1-AT levels compared to controls have been described in adult patients with acute ischemic heart disease [32]. Another study that should be mentioned here is the study of Dahl et al. [33], who observed that α_1-AT deficiency caused by *MZ* heterozygosity is associated with a reduced risk of ischemic cerebrovascular disease and ischemic heart disease. Thus, if a low concentration of α_1-AT reduces the risk of ischemic vascular disease, then vice versa this would support the hypothesis that an increased α_1-AT level is a risk factor for IS. In agreement with these findings Espana et al. [34] demonstrated that the APC:α_1-AT complex can be used as a sensitive marker of prothrombotic states.

In contributing to the risk of pediatric thromboembolism the importance of various hereditary hemostatic abnormalities is well established [35]. To date, the rate of single or combined prothrombotic risk factors detected in Caucasian children is approximately 50%, while no thrombophilia has been found in the remaining subjects [12, 14, 17, 36]. Data presented here give evidence that increased α_1-AT concentrations greater than age-dependent 90th percentiles further contribute as a significant and independent risk factor to symptomatic IS in Caucasian children, in 17.3% of cases not combined with one of the established risk factors. The OR found was 4.0 for subjects with thromboembolic stroke, i.e. clearly within the range reported for further inherited thrombophilic risk factors in white children, e.g. the heterozygous FV G1691A mutation, the FII G20210A variant or elevated Lp(a) levels.

The results shown here, indicating that α_1-AT concentrations greater than age-dependent 90th percentiles are a risk factor for stroke in children, are in accordance with the majority of findings in adults. However, since the blood used to determine the α_1-AT level had not been drawn until well after the onset of the acute stroke it is unlikely that the elevation in the α_1-AT level could have been caused by the stroke itself. Along with normal values for fibrinogen, D-dimer and prothrombin fragment F1.2 at the time of evaluation (data not shown) we suggest that elevation of α_1-AT is more likely a cause rather than a consequence of the stroke event. In addition, since the 1980s information has been available that there are important physiological differences in the hemostatic system in children compared with adults [20]. In contrast to lower levels of the natural anticoagulant inhibitors protein C and protein S in early childhood, α_2-macroglobulin and C1-inactivator are elevated until puberty [20, 37], and α_1-AT concentrations as earlier reported and established in the healthy cohort investigated here are lower beyond the neonatal period in the first year of life and increase in infants and children during puberty [20, 38, 39]. As a consequence in the last 20 years the need for age-dependent normal values to correctly classify bleeding as well as thrombotic tendencies in neonates, infants and children has increasingly been accepted and normal age-dependent values should be applied when conducting risk assessment studies in children.

In summary, besides the established risk factors, an α_1-AT concentration greater than the 90th age-dependent percentiles is another risk factor for stroke in Caucasian children, increasing the laboratory rate of detecting risk factors not combined with established thrombophilic risks in 17% of patients. However, the findings of the present study are restricted to white German stroke children, and further studies are recommended to clarify the role of increased α_1-AT in pediatric populations not of Caucasian origin. In addition, further longitudinal follow-up studies are necessary to better evaluate and understand the role of α_1-AT during the acute and nonacute phase following arterial thromboembolism.

Acknowledgements

This study was supported by unrestricted grants of the Karl-Bröcker-Stiftung. We thank Kai Griesbach for editing the manuscript.

References

1 Andrew M, David M, Adams M, Ali K, Anderson R, Barnard D, Bernstein M, Brisson L, Cairney B, DeSai D, Grant R, Israels S, Jardine L, Luke B, Massciotte P, Silva M: Venous thromboembolic complications (VTE) in children: first analyses of the Canadian registry of VTE. Blood 1994;83:1251–1257.
2 Lynch JK: Cerebrovascular disorders in children. Curr Neurol Neurosci Rep 2004;4:129–138.
3 Andrew M: Developmental hemostasis: relevance to thromboembolic complications in pediatric patients. Thromb Haemost 1995;74:415–425.
4 Schmidt B, Andrew M: Neonatal thrombosis: report of a prospective Canadian and international registry. Pediatrics 1995;96:939–943.
5 Massicotte MP, Dix D, Monagle P, Adams M, Andrew M: Central venous catheter related thrombosis in children: analysis of the Canadian Registry of venous thromboembolic complications. J Pediatr 1998;133:770–776.
6 Monagle P, Adams M, Mahoney M, Ali K, Barnard D, Bernstein M, Brisson L, David M, Desai S, Scully MF, Halton J, Israels S, Jardine L, Leaker M, McCusker P, Silva M, Wu J, Anderson R, Andrew M, Massciotte MP: Outcome of pediatric thromboembolic disease: a report from the Canadian childhood thrombophilia registry. Pediatr Res 2000;47:763–766.
7 Van Ommen CH, Heijboer H, Buller HR, Hirasing RA, Heijmans HS, Peters M: Venous thromboembolism in childhood: a prospective two-year registry in The Netherlands. J Pediatr 2001;139:676–681.
8 de Stefano V, Finazzi G, Mannucci PM: Inherited thrombophilia: pathogenesis, clinical syndromes and management. Blood 1996;87:3531–3544.
9 Lane DA, Mannucci PM, Bauer KA, Bertina RM, Bochkov NP, Boulyjenkov V, Chandy M, Dahlbäck B, Ginter EK, Miletich JP, Rosendaal FR, Seligsohn U: Inherited thrombophilia. Part I. Thromb Haemost 1996;76:651–662.
10 Lane DA, Mannucci PM, Bauer KA, Bertina RM, Bochkov NP, Boulyjenkov V, Chandy M, Dahlbäck B, Ginter EK, Miletich JP, Rosendaal FR, Seligsohn U: Inherited thrombophilia. Part II. Thromb Haemost 1996;76:824–834.
11 Poort SR, Rosendaal FR, Reitsma PH, Bertina RM: A common genetic variation in the 3′-untranslated region of the prothrombin gene is associated with elevated plasma prothrombin levels and an increase in venous thrombosis. Blood 1996;88:3698–3703.
12 Junker R, Koch HG, Auberger K, Münchow N, Ehrenforth S, Nowak-Göttl U: Prothrombin G20210A gene mutation and further prothrombotic risk factors in childhood thrombophilia. Arterioscler Thromb Vasc Biol 1999;19:2568–2572.
13 Kosch A, Koch HG, Heinecke A, Kurnik K, Heller C, Nowak-Göttl U; Childhood Thrombophilia Study Group: Increased fasting total homocysteine plasma levels as a risk factor for thromboembolism in children. Thromb Haemost 2004;91:308–314.
14 Nowak-Göttl U, Junker R, Hartmeier M, Koch HG, Münchow N, Assmann G, von Eckardstein A: Increased lipoprotein(a) is an important risk factor for venous thromboembolism in childhood. Circulation 1999;100:743–748.
15 Heeb MJ, Griffin JH: Physiologic inhibition of human activated protein C by α1-antitrypsin. J Biol Chem 1988;263:11613–11616.
16 van der Meer FJ, van Tilburg NH, van Wijngaarden A, van der Linden IK, Briet E, Bertina RM: A second plasma inhibitor of activated protein C: alpha 1-antitrypsin. Thromb Haemost 1989;62:756–762.
17 Nowak-Göttl U, Sträter R, Heinecke A, Junker R, Koch HG, Schuierer G, von Eckardstein A: Lipoprotein (a) and genetic polymorphisms of clotting factor V, prothrombin, and methylenetetrahydrofolate reductase are risk factors of spontaneous ischemic stroke in childhood. Blood 1999;94:3678–3682.
18 Andrew M, Paes B, Milner R, Johnston M, Mitchell L, Tollefsen DM, Powers P: Development of the human coagulation system in the full-term infant. Blood 1987;70:165–172.
19 Andrew M, Paes B, Johnston M: Development of the hemostatic system in the neonate and young infant. Clinical research update. Am J Pediatr Hematol Oncol 1990;12:95–104.
20 Andrew M, Vegh P, Johnston M, Bowker J, Ofosu F, Mitchell L: Maturation of the hemostatic system during childhood. Blood 1992;80:1998–2005.
21 Pratt CW, Church FC: General features of the heparin-binding serpins antithrombin, heparin cofactor II and protein C inhibitor. Blood Coagul Fibrinolysis 1993;4:479–490.
22 Sakata Y, Loskutoff DJ, Gladson CL, Hekman CM, Griffin JH: Mechanism of protein C-dependent clot lysis: role of plasminogen activator inhibitor. Blood 1986;68:1218–1223.
23 Bruch M, Weiss V, Engel J: Plasma serine proteinase inhibitors (serpins) exhibit major conformational changes and a large increase in conformational stability upon cleavage at their reactive sites. J Biol Chem 1988;263:16626–16630.
24 Gettins P, Patston PA, Schapira M: Structure and mechanism of action of serpins. Hematol Oncol Clin North Am 1992;6:1393–1408.
25 Whisstock J, Skinner R, Lesk AM: An atlas of serpin conformations. Trends Biochem Sci 1998;23:63–67.
26 Rezaie AR: Exosite-dependent regulation of the protein C anticoagulant pathway. Trends Cardiovasc Med 2003;13:8–15.
27 Heeb MJ, Mosher DF, Griffin JH: Activation and complexation of protein C and cleavage and decrease of protein S in plasma of patients with intravascular coagulation. Blood 1989;73:455–461.
28 Marlar RA, Kressin DC, Madden RM: Contribution of plasma proteinase inhibitors to the regulation of activated protein C in plasma. Thromb Haemost 1993;69:16–20.

29 Espana F, Gruber A, Heeb MJ, Hanson SR, Harker LA, Griffin JH: In vivo and in vitro complexes of activated protein C with two inhibitors in baboons. Blood 1991;77:1754–1760.
30 Fletcher AP, Alkjaersig N, Davies A, Lewis M, Brooks J, Hardin W, Landau W, Raichle ME: Blood coagulation and plasma fibrinolytic enzyme system pathophysiology in stroke. Stroke 1976;7:337–348.
31 Bartosik-Psujek H, Belniak E, Stelmasiak Z: Markers of inflammation in cerebral ischemia. Neurol Sci 2003;24:279–280.
32 Losito R, Gattiker H, Bilodeau G, Verville N, Longpre B: Levels of antithrombin III, alpha 2-macroglobulin, and alpha 1-antitrypsin in acute ischemic heart disease. J Lab Clin Med 1981;97:241–250.
33 Dahl M, Tybjaerg-Hansen A, Sillesen H, Jensen G, Steffensen R, Nordestgaard BG: Blood pressure, risk of ischemic cerebrovascular and ischemic heart disease, and longevity in B1-antitrypsin deficiency. Circulation 2003;107: 747–752.
34 Espana F, Gilabert J, Vicente V, Estelles A, Vazquez L, Hendl S, Aznar J: Activated protein C:alpha 1-antitrypsin (APC:alpha 1 AT) complex as a marker for in vitro diagnosis of prethrombotic state. Thromb Res 1992;66: 499–508.
35 Lane A, Grant PJ: Role of hemostatic gene polymorphisms in venous and arterial thrombotic disease. Blood 2000;95:1517–1526.
36 Bonduel M, Hepner M, Sciuccati G, Torres AF, Pieroni G, Frontroth JP: Prothrombotic abnormalities in children with venous thromboembolism. J Pediatr Hematol Oncol 2000; 22:66–72.
37 Ehrenforth S, Junker R, Koch HG, Kreuz W, Muenchow N, Scharrer I, Nowak-Goettl U: Multicentre evaluation of combined prothrombotic defects associated with thrombophilia in childhood. Eur J Pediatr 1999;158:S97–S104.
38 Ward AM, White PA, Wild G: Reference ranges for serum alpha 1 antitrypsin. Arch Dis Child 1985;60:261–262.
39 Lockitch G, Halstead AC, Quigley G, MacCallum C: Age- and sex-specific pediatric reference intervals: study design and methods illustrated by measurement of serum proteins with the Behring LN Nephelometer. Clin Chem 1988;34:1618–1621.

Acta Haematologica

Acta Haematol 2006;115:192–197
DOI: 10.1159/000090934

3′ End Processing of the Prothrombin mRNA in Thrombophilia

Sven Danckwardt[a, b] Kathrin Hartmann[a, b] Niels H. Gehring[a, b]
Matthias W. Hentze[b, c] Andreas E. Kulozik[a, b]

[a]Department of Pediatric Oncology, Hematology and Immunology, University of Heidelberg,
[b]EMBL – University of Heidelberg Molecular Medicine Partnership Unit,
[c]European Molecular Biology Laboratory, Heidelberg, Germany

Key Words

F2 20210*A · F2 20221*T mutation · mRNA processing · Polyadenylation · Thrombophilia

Abstract

Clinical and genetic studies have led to the discovery of specific genotypes that predispose to thromboembolism in adults and children. The exploration of the underlying pathologies has revealed a broad variety of affected molecular mechanisms. Most recently, the functional analysis of the prothrombin (F2) 20210*A variant revealed increased efficiency of 3′ end processing as a novel genetic mechanism predisposing to human disease. Here, we review the 3′ end processing of the human F2 mRNA and demonstrate how clinically relevant mutations in the F2 gene contribute to thrombophilia by interfering with a tightly balanced architecture of noncanonical 3′ end formation signals.

Introduction

Venous thrombosis occurs in about 1:1,000 people in developed countries each year. Although increasingly diagnosed, thromboses during childhood are still a rare event with an incidence of ~0.01% [1] in comparison to an estimated incidence of 2.5–5% in adults [2]. The incidence of thrombosis is strongly dependent on age and increases during lifetime [3], which reflects both, the acquisition of environmental risk factors and the development of pro- and anticoagulatory enzymes and the fibrinolytic system during childhood and adolescence [4]. Several factors that predispose to thrombosis are well established. Among the acquired conditions, acute and chronic diseases, vascular interventions, bone surgery, immobilization and drugs frequently act together with inherited genetic risk factors, which finally results in thrombosis. The multifactorial nature of thrombosis is especially apparent in children who often display multiple risk factors at the time of diagnosis [1, 5]. The presence of a central venous line plays a particularly important role in children and has been shown to be associated with up to 60% of pediatric thrombosis and up to 90% in newborns [3, 6–8]. Among the inherited risk factors, the FV Leiden mutation and an elevated lipoprotein (a) play important roles both prenatally and in childhood [9, 10].

Under physiological conditions, blood coagulation is a tightly controlled process that is controlled by fail-safe mechanisms to maintain hemostasis and to prevent intravascular thrombosis and embolism. In particular, thrombin plays a key role in the regulation of the blood coagulation cascade. It acts as a procoagulant enzyme by activating factors XI, VIII, V and the thrombin-activat-

KARGER
Fax +41 61 306 12 34
E-Mail karger@karger.ch
www.karger.com

0001–5792/06/1154–0192$23.50/0

Accessible online at:
www.karger.com/aha

Andreas E. Kulozik
Molecular Medicine Partnership Unit, Im Neuenheimer Feld 153
DE–69120 Heidelberg (Germany)
Tel. +49 6221 564555, Fax +49 6221 564559
E-Mail Andreas.Kulozik@med.uni-heidelberg.de

able fibrinolysis inhibitor and by cleaving fibrinogen to release fibrin, the major component of blood clots. Moreover, thrombin also acts as an anticoagulant enzyme by activating protein C [11]. The pivotal role of thrombin in the regulation of hemostasis is illustrated by the identification of the common F2 20210*A allele. This mutation causes raised prothrombin plasma concentrations and predisposes carriers to develop thromboses [12–15]. The F2 20210*A allele is found in approximately 2% of the white Caucasian population, although there are regional differences [16]. However, among adult patients with thrombosis the prevalence of this mutation is 6%, which reflects a ~3-fold increased risk for developing thrombosis in heterozygotes and a ~20-fold increased risk in homozygously affected individuals. The underlying molecular mechanism of F2 20210*A has previously been identified to represent enhanced 3′ end formation as a novel principle resulting in human disease [17]. This emphasizes that even (minor) changes in mRNA maturation such as 3′ end processing can have deleterious effects (see below).

3′ End Processing and Prothrombin Mutations in Thrombophilia

Physiologically, the specificity and efficiency of 3′ end processing is determined by the binding of a multiprotein complex to the 3′ end processing signal [18, 19]. Most pre-mRNAs contain two core sequence elements (fig. 1). The canonical polyadenylation signal AAUAAA upstream of the cleavage site is recognized by the multimeric cleavage/polyadenylation specificity factor (CPSF). This RNA-protein interaction determines the site of cleavage 10–30 nt downstream, preferentially immediately 3′ of a CA dinucleotide [20]. The second canonical sequence element is characterized by a high density of G/U or U residues and is located up to 30 nt downstream of the cleavage site. This sequence element is bound by the 64-kDa subunit of the heterotrimeric cleavage-stimulating factor (CstF) that promotes the efficiency of 3′ end processing. Both of these multimeric protein complexes are of special importance; they travel with the RNA polymerase II (Pol II) C-terminal domain (CTD) during transcription and are transferred to their specific 3′ end processing signals on the RNA molecule as it emerges from the RNA polymerase. Additional proteins, cleavage factor I and II (CFI, CFII), associate and the pre-mRNA is cleaved. Subsequently, the poly(A) polymerase (PAP) adds ~200 A nucleotides to the 3′ end in a template-independent manner. Finally, several molecules of the poly(A)-binding protein II (PAB II) bind to the poly(A) residues and determine the length of the poly(A) tail. These proteins remain attached at the poly(A) tail during nuclear export and enhance both, the stability and the translation of the mRNA [for a review, see 21]. Therefore, defects of mRNA 3′ end formation can profoundly alter cell viability, growth, and development by interfering with well-coordinated cellular processes.

The medical relevance of errors of 3′ end processing is exemplified by mutations of the highly conserved polyadenylation signal (AAUAAA) which invariably inactivate gene expression causing a variety of diseases [22–32]. Moreover, depletion of the 64-kDa subunit of CstF can lead to cell cycle arrest and affect apoptosis [33], and a defective poly(A) polymerase regulation causes cell accumulation in the G0-G1 phase [34]. Consistent with these observations the cell cycle-regulated poly(A) polymerase activity [35] has been suggested to reflect the proliferative activity of cells, and thus might serve as a prognostic factor in cancer [for a review, see 36, 37]. Furthermore, a loss-of-function mutation of the PAB II has been shown to be associated with oculopharyngeal muscular dystrophy [38], which further illustrates the medical importance of intact *trans*-acting factors in 3′ end processing.

Inasmuch as very little is known about mutations that affect 3′ end processing the elucidation of the molecular mechanism of the common F2 20210*A variant is particularly intriguing. This mutation is located in the F2 3′ untranslated region and affects the most 3′ nucleotide where the pre-mRNA is endonucleolytically cleaved and polyadenylated [17]. It is noteworthy that physiological 3′ cleavage of the wild-type F2 mRNA occurs 3′ of a CG dinucleotide, whereas most mRNAs are cleaved 3′ of a CA dinucleotide. The CG dinucleotide has been shown to be less efficient in promoting the cleavage reaction in vitro [20] and the CG→CA mutation at the cleavage site increases 3′ end processing efficiency in cell lines and in transgenic mice [17, 39]. Hence, the G→A mutation at position 20210 reverts the physiologically inefficient F2 cleavage site into the most favorable CA dinucleotide context: it increases cleavage site recognition and results in the accumulation of correctly 3′ end processed and translatable prothrombin mRNA in the cytoplasm. In addition, F2 20210*A may also enhance translation efficiency due to a change in the location of the 3′ end cleavage/polyadenylation reaction [40]. Enhanced mRNA 3′ end formation efficiency thus emerges as a novel molecular principle causing pathological gene expression and explains the role of F2 20210*A in the pathogenesis of thrombophilia.

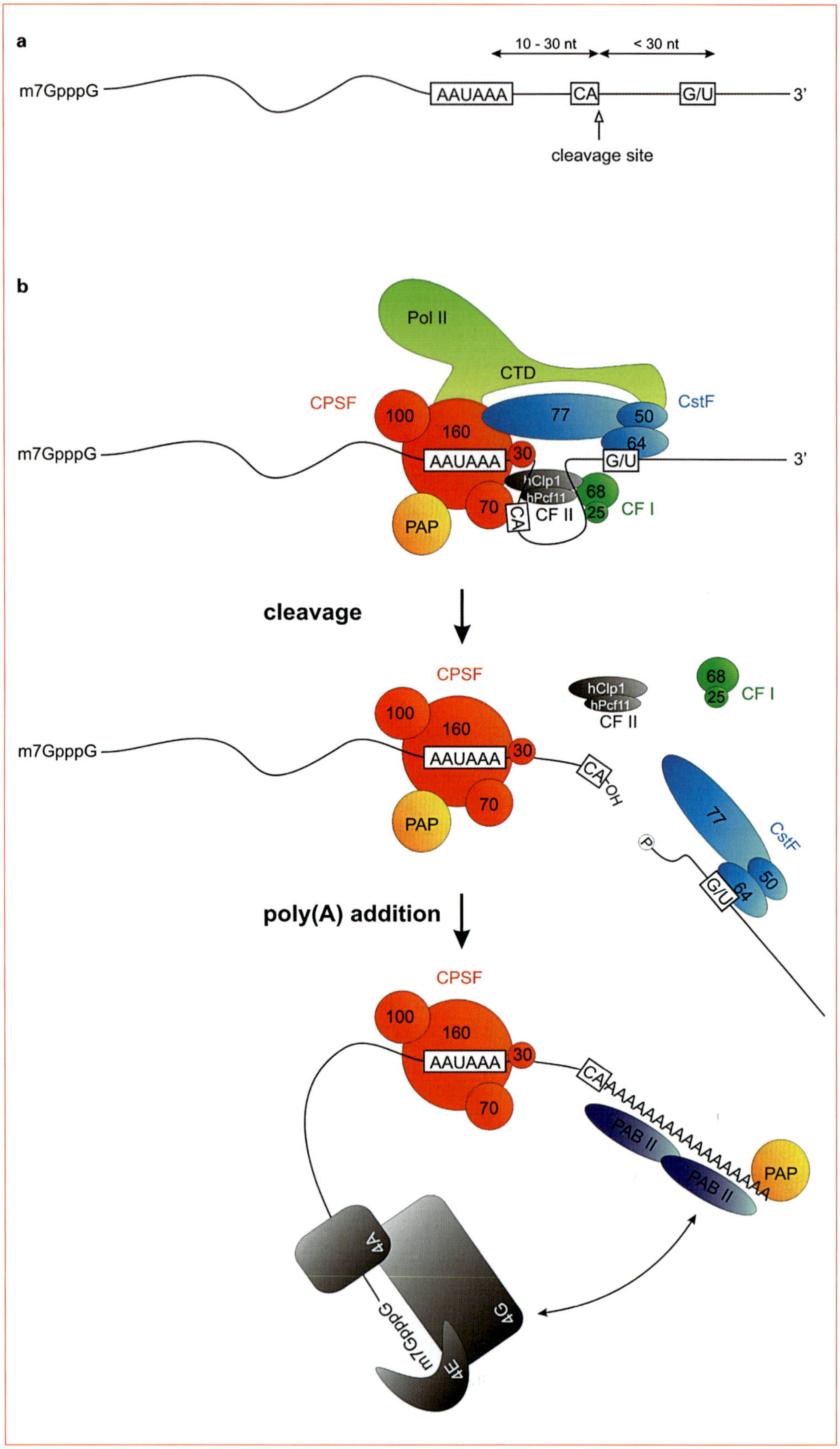

Fig. 1. *Cis*-acting sequence elements and *trans*-acting factors involved in mammalian 3′ end processing. **a** Schematic representation of the (obligatory) *cis*-acting determinants of mammalian poly(A) signals. The hexanucleotide AAUAAA [poly(A) signal] is located 10–30 nt upstream of the cleavage site CA dinucleotide. A G/U- or U-rich region is located up to 30 nt downstream of the cleavage site. **b** mRNA precursors are processed at their 3′ ends. After the assembly of a multiprotein complex, the primary transcript is endonucleolytically cleaved at the cleavage site. This is followed by the addition of adenine residues to the 3′ end to form a poly(A) tail which is bound by PAB II that establish contact to the translation initiation factor eIF4G as part of the initiation complex, thus generating a translation-competent ribonucleoprotein particle. CstF = Cleavage-stimulating factor (blue complex); CPSF = cleavage/polyadenylation specificity factor (red complex); Pol II = RNA polymerase II (light green complex) with C-terminal domain (CTD); CF I = cleavage factor I (green complex); CF II = cleavage factor II (grey complex); PAP = poly(A) polymerase (yellow complex); PAB II = poly(A)-binding proteins II (dark blue complex); 4A, 4E, 4G = translation initiation factors (grey complex).

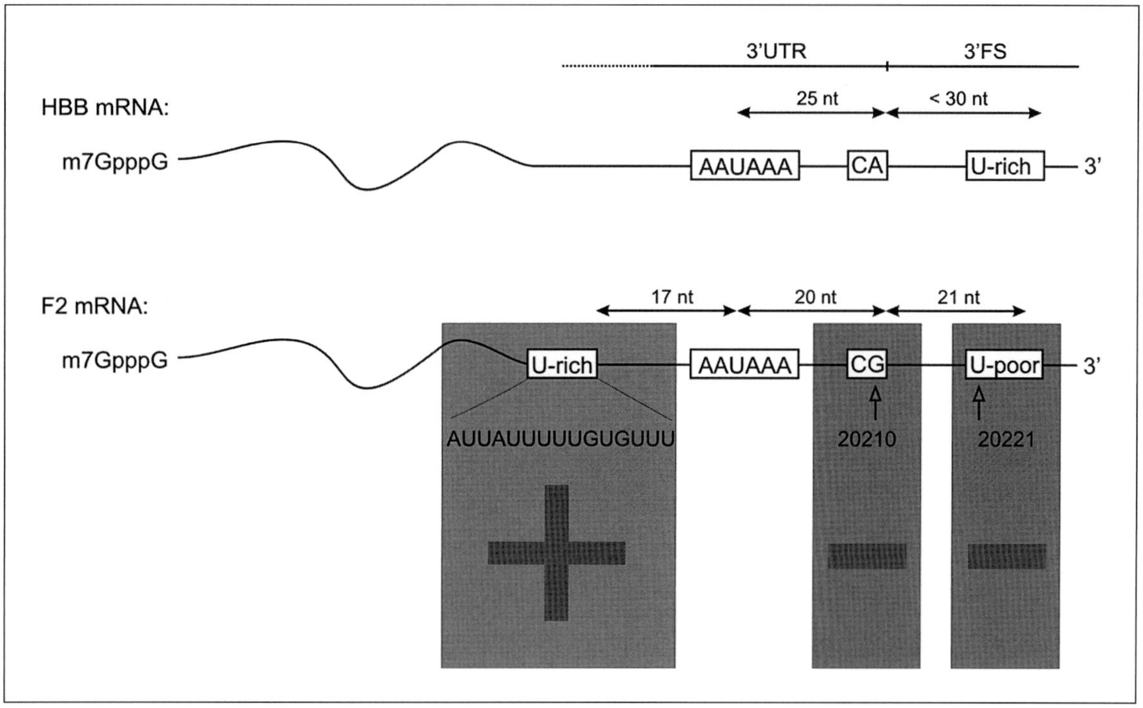

Fig. 2. The human prothrombin 3′ end processing signal shows an unusual architecture of noncanonical sequence elements which are susceptible to gain-of-function mutations. A sequence comparison of the 3′ end processing signals of efficiently processed mRNAs such as SV40 late or β-globin (HBB, upper lane) with prothrombin (F2, lower lane) revealed an inefficient F2 cleavage dinucleotide context and an uridine-poor downstream element. In contrast, the F2 3′ untranslated region contains a uridine-rich upstream element that promotes 3′ end processing and, hence, balances F2 mRNA expression. 3′ UTR = 3′ Untranslated region; 3′ FS = 3′ flanking sequence; AAUAAA = polyadenylation signal.

Recently, further attention has been attracted by the report of a novel disease related F2 mutation 11 nucleotides downstream of the cleavage site. This novel C→T mutation at position 20221 (F2 20221*T) has been identified in a 9-year-old patient with an acute vascular rejection and intrarenal segmental arterial thrombosis of an allogeneic kidney transplant [41], in a 28-year-old man with Budd-Chiari syndrome [42], and has also been found to be associated with recurrent fetal loss and intrauterine growth retardation in a 40-year-old South Asian female with a family history of thrombosis [43]. Although this rare mutation has only been found in a small number of patients, the location in the F2 3′ end processing signal and the observed clinical phenotypes suggest that the F2 20221 mutation may be thrombosis related by increasing 3′ end processing efficiency. A recent systematic analysis of F2 3′ end formation determinants identified an unusual architecture of noncanonical sequence elements that explains the susceptibility of the F2 3′ end processing region to gain-of-function mutations (fig. 2). (1) The F2 3′ end formation signal contains the least efficient dinucleotide context at the physiological cleavage site (CG instead of CA). (2) The F2 (downstream) U-rich element has been found to be uridine-poor compared to efficiently 3′ end processed mRNAs such as β-globin (HBB) and SV40. Consequently, the introduction of (an) additional uridine residue(s) in the F2 3′ flanking sequence by either the novel F2 20221*T mutation or by an experimental insertion at adjacent sites enhances 3′ end processing, presumably by facilitating the CstF-mRNA interaction (see above). (3) The F2 3′ untranslated region contains a stimulatory (upstream) U-rich element that appears to compensate for the weak functional activities of the cleavage site and the (downstream) U-rich element in the F2 3′ flanking sequence. The F2 3′ end processing signal thus appears to be balanced by an unusual architecture of weak and stimulatory sequence elements [44].

The biological impact of this unconventional composition of the F2 3′ end processing signal has not yet been elucidated, and it is tempting to speculate that 3′ end for-

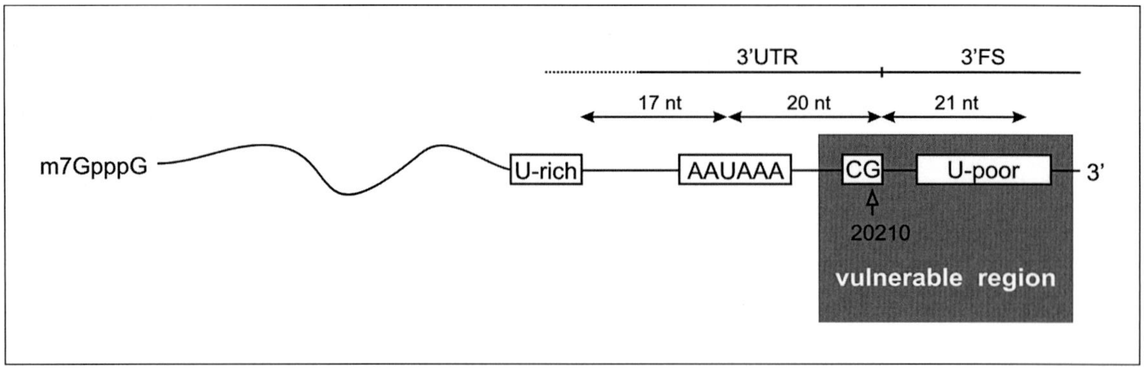

Fig. 3. The human prothrombin gene contains a 'vulnerable region' for gain-of-function mutations encompassing the cleavage site and the 3′ flanking sequence (3′FS).

mation of this mRNA might be differentially regulated [34, 45–47]. The unusual architecture of the F2 3′ end processing signal gains medical significance because it creates a 'vulnerable region' encompassing the entire cleavage site including the 3′ flanking sequence in which N→T transitions may give rise to clinically relevant gain-of-function phenotypes (fig. 3). This prediction becomes even more evident taking into consideration that other – albeit experimentally introduced – mutations within the F2 cleavage site and the 3′ flanking sequence have already been shown to result in marked upregulation of F2 mRNA expression [44]. Bearing this in mind, a complete diagnostic workup for unexplained thrombophilia may have to include DNA sequence analysis of the F2 3′ end processing region and the identification of the F2 20210*A allele alone may not be sufficient.

Acknowledgments

This work was supported by the Deutsche Forschungsgesellschaft (DFG) and the DFG Forschergruppe (FOR 426): Complex RNA-Protein Interactions in the Maturation and Function of Eukaryotic mRNA. We thank Frau Margit Pförsich for technical assistance.

References

1 Andrew M, David M, Adams M, Ali K, Anderson R, Barnard D, Bernstein M, Brisson L, Cairney B, DeSai D, Grant R, Israels S, Jardine L, Luke B, Massicotte P, Silva M: Venous thromboembolic complications (VTE) in children: first analyses of the Canadian Registry of VTE. Blood 1994;83:1251–1257.
2 Weinmann EE, Salzman EW: Deep-vein thrombosis. N Engl J Med 1994;331:1630–1641.
3 Rosendaal FR: Thrombosis in the young: epidemiology and risk factors. A focus on venous thrombosis. Thromb Haemost 1997;78:1–6.
4 Richardson MW, Allen GA, Monahan PE: Thrombosis in children: current perspective and distinct challenges. Thromb Haemost 2002;88:900–911.
5 Rosendaal FR: Venous thrombosis: a multicausal disease. Lancet 1999;353:1167–1173.
6 Nowak-Gottl U, Kosch A, Schlegel N, Salem M, Manco-Johnson M: Thromboembolism in children. Curr Opin Hematol 2002;9:448–453.
7 Massicotte MP, Dix D, Monagle P, Adams M, Andrew M: Central venous catheter related thrombosis in children: analysis of the Canadian Registry of Venous Thromboembolic Complications. J Pediatr 1998;133:770–776.
8 Schmidt B, Andrew M: Neonatal thrombosis: report of a prospective Canadian and international registry. Pediatrics 1995;96:939–943.
9 Hundsdoerfer P, Vetter B, Stover B, Bassir C, Scholz T, Grimmer I, Monch E, Ziemer S, Rossi R, Kulozik AE: Homozygous and double heterozygous factor V Leiden and factor II G20210A genotypes predispose infants to thromboembolism but are not associated with an increase of foetal loss. Thromb Haemost 2003;90:628–635.
10 Kosch A, Kuwertz-Broking E, Heller C, Kurnik K, Schobess R, Nowak-Gottl U: Renal venous thrombosis in neonates: prothrombotic risk factors and long-term follow-up. Blood 2004;104:1356–1360.
11 Dahlback B: Blood coagulation. Lancet 2000;355:1627–1632.
12 Poort SR, Rosendaal FR, Reitsma PH, Bertina RM: A common genetic variation in the 3′-untranslated region of the prothrombin gene is associated with elevated plasma prothrombin levels and an increase in venous thrombosis. Blood 1996;88:3698–3703.
13 Cattaneo M, Chantarangkul V, Taioli E, Santos JH, Tagliabue L: The G20210A mutation of the prothrombin gene in patients with previous first episodes of deep-vein thrombosis: prevalence and association with factor V G1691A, methylenetetrahydrofolate reductase C677T and plasma prothrombin levels. Thromb Res 1999;93:1–8.
14 Makris M, Preston FE, Beauchamp NJ, Cooper PC, Daly ME, Hampton KK, Bayliss P, Peake IR, Miller GJ: Co-inheritance of the 20210A allele of the prothrombin gene increases the risk of thrombosis in subjects with familial thrombophilia. Thromb Haemost 1997;78:1426–1429.

15 Soria JM, Almasy L, Souto JC, Tirado I, Borell M, Mateo J, Slifer S, Stone W, Blangero J, Fontcuberta J: Linkage analysis demonstrates that the prothrombin G20210A mutation jointly influences plasma prothrombin levels and risk of thrombosis. Blood 2000;95:2780–2785.
16 Rosendaal FR, Doggen CJ, Zivelin A, Arruda VR, Aiach M, Siscovick DS, Hillarp A, Watzke HH, Bernardi F, Cumming AM, Preston FE, Reitsma PH: Geographic distribution of the 20210 G to A prothrombin variant. Thromb Haemost 1998;79:706–708.
17 Gehring NH, Frede U, Neu-Yilik G, Hundsdoerfer P, Vetter B, Hentze MW, Kulozik AE: Increased efficiency of mRNA 3′ end formation: a new genetic mechanism contributing to hereditary thrombophilia. Nat Genet 2001;28: 389–392.
18 Colgan DF, Manley JL: Mechanism and regulation of mRNA polyadenylation. Genes Dev 1997;11:2755–2766.
19 Keller W, Minvielle-Sebastia L: A comparison of mammalian and yeast premRNA 3′-end processing. Curr Opin Cell Biol 1997;9:329–336.
20 Chen F, MacDonald CC, Wilusz J: Cleavage site determinants in the mammalian polyadenylation signal. Nucleic Acids Res 1995;23: 2614–2620.
21 Zhao J, Hyman L, Moore C: Formation of mRNA 3′ ends in eukaryotes: mechanism, regulation, and interrelationships with other steps in mRNA synthesis. Microbiol Mol Biol Rev 1999;63:405–445.
22 Higgs DR, Goodbourn SE, Lamb J, Clegg JB, Weatherall DJ, Proudfoot NJ: Alpha-thalassaemia caused by a polyadenylation signal mutation. Nature 1983;306:398–400.
23 Orkin SH, Cheng TC, Antonarakis SE, Kazazian HH Jr: Thalassemia due to a mutation in the cleavage-polyadenylation signal of the human beta-globin gene. EMBO J 1985;4:453–456.
24 Jankovic L, Efremov GD, Petkov G, Kattamis C, George E, Yang KG, Stoming TA, Huisman TH: Two novel polyadenylation mutations leading to beta(+)-thalassemia. Br J Haematol 1990;75:122–126.
25 Rund D, Dowling C, Najjar K, Rachmilewitz E, Kazazian H Jr, Oppenheim A: Two mutations in the (beta)-globin polyadenylylation signal reveal extended transcripts and new RNA polyadenylylation sites. Proc Natl Acad Sci USA 1992;89:4324–4328.
26 Harteveld CL, Losekoot M, Haak H, Heister GA, Giordano PC, Bernini LF: A novel polyadenylation signal mutation in the alpha 2-globin gene causing alpha thalassaemia. Br J Haematol 1994;87:139–143.
27 van Solinge WW, Lind B, van Wijk R, Hart HC, Kraaijenhagen RJ: Clinical expression of a rare beta-globin gene mutation co-inherited with haemoglobin E-disease. Eur J Clin Chem Clin Biochem 1996;34:949–954.
28 Gieselmann V, Polten A, Kreysing J, von Figura K: Arylsulfatase A pseudodeficiency: loss of a polyadenylylation signal and N-glycosylation site. Proc Natl Acad Sci USA 1989;86: 9436–9440.
29 Barth ML, Fensom A, Harris A: Prevalence of common mutations in the arylsulphatase A gene in metachromatic leukodystrophy patients diagnosed in Britain. Hum Genet 1993; 91:73–77.
30 Harvey J, Carey W, Morris C: Importance of the glycosylation and polyadenylation variants in metachromatic leukodystrophy pseudodeficiency phenotype. Hum Mol Genet 1998;7: 1215–1219.
31 Bell DA, Stephens EA, Castranio T, Umbach DM, Watson M, Deakin M, Elder J, Hendrickse C, Duncan H, Strange RC: Polyadenylation polymorphism in the acetyltransferase 1 gene (NAT1) increases risk of colorectal cancer. Cancer Res 1995;55:3537–3542.
32 Kleiman FE, Manley JL: Functional interaction of BRCA1-associated BARD1 with polyadenylation factor CstF-50. Science 1999;285: 1576–1579.
33 Takagaki Y, Manley JL: Levels of polyadenylation factor CstF-64 control IgM heavy chain mRNA accumulation and other events associated with B cell differentiation. Mol Cell 1998; 2:761–771.
34 Zhao W, Manley JL: Complex alternative RNA processing generates an unexpected diversity of poly(A) polymerase isoforms. Mol Cell Biol 1996;16:2378–2386.
35 Colgan DF, Murthy KG, Prives C, Manley JL: Cell-cycle related regulation of poly(A) polymerase by phosphorylation. Nature 1996;384: 282–285.
36 Jacob ST, Terns MP, Maguire KA: Polyadenylate polymerases from normal and cancer cells and their potential role in messenger RNA processing: a review. Cancer Res 1989;49:2827–2833.
37 Scorilas A: Polyadenylate polymerase (PAP) and 3′ end pre-mRNA processing: function, assays, and association with disease. Crit Rev Clin Lab Sci 2002;39:193–224.
38 Brais B, Bouchard JP, Xie YG, Rochefort DL, Chretien N, Tome FM, Lafreniere RG, Rommens JM, Uyama E, Nohira O, Blumen S, Korczyn AD, Heutink P, Mathieu J, Duranceau A, Codere F, Fardeau M, Rouleau GA: Short GCG expansions in the PABP2 gene cause oculopharyngeal muscular dystrophy. Nat Genet 1998;18:164–167.
39 Kuwahara M, Kurachi S, Kurachi K: Molecular mechanism of prothrombin G20210A variant: critical new role of exon splicing enhancer in poly (A) tailing. Blood 2004;104:abstract 1944.
40 Pollak ES, Lam HS, Russell JE: The G20210A mutation does not affect the stability of prothrombin mRNA in vivo. Blood 2002;100: 359–362.
41 Wylenzek M, Geisen C, Stapenhorst L, Wielckens K, Klingler KR: A novel point mutation in the 3′ region of the prothrombin gene at position 20221 in a Lebanese/Syrian family. Thromb Haemost 2001;85:943–944.
42 Balim Z, Kosova B, Falzon K, Bezzina Wettinger S, Colak Y: Budd-Chiari syndrome in a patient heterozygous for the point mutation C20221T of the prothrombin gene. J Thromb Haemost 2003;1:852–853.
43 Schrijver I, Lenzi TJ, Jones CD, Lay MJ, Druzin ML, Zehnder JL: Prothrombin gene variants in non-Caucasians with fetal loss and intrauterine growth retardation. J Mol Diagn 2003;5:250–253.
44 Danckwardt S, Gehring NH, Neu-Yilik G, Hundsdoerfer P, Pforsich M, Frede U, Hentze MW, Kulozik AE: The prothrombin 3′ end formation signal reveals a unique architecture that is sensitive to thrombophilic gain-of-function mutations. Blood 2004;104:428–435.
45 Lou H, Gagel RF: Alternative RNA processing – its role in regulating expression of calcitonin/calcitonin gene-related peptide. J Endocrinol 1998;156:401–405.
46 Barabino SM, Keller W: Last but not least: regulated poly(A) tail formation. Cell 1999;99: 9–11.
47 Edwalds-Gilbert G, Veraldi KL, Milcarek C: Alternative poly(A) site selection in complex transcription units: means to an end? Nucleic Acids Res 1997;25:2547–2561.

Acta Haematologica

Acta Haematol 2006;115:198–200
DOI: 10.1159/000090935

Venous Thromboembolism after Severe Injury in Children

Claude Cyr[a] Bruno Michon[b] Géraldine Pettersen[a] Michèle David[b]
Josée Brossard[a]

[a]Département de pédiatrie, Faculté de Médecine, Université de Sherbrooke et [b]Service d'hématologie, Hopital Sainte-Justine, Montréal, Canada

Key Words
Injury · Thrombosis · Venous thromboembolism

Abstract

Background: Deep vein thrombosis and pulmonary embolism are considered common complications after major trauma. Their incidence and the associated risk factors have rarely been identified in injured children. ***Methods:*** Severely injured children (age <18 years; admitted in a pediatric intensive care unit or length of stay ≥72 h) with a discharge diagnosis of venous thromboembolism (VTE; deep venous thrombosis and/or pulmonary embolism) were identified from the institutional trauma registry between January 1, 1999 and April 31, 2002. The study centers included a dedicated pediatric trauma center and an adult trauma center with pediatric patients. Risk factors for VTE were identified using multivariate analysis. ***Results:*** VTE was found in 11 of the 3,291 admissions, for a rate of 3.3/1,000 admissions. Children with VTE were older and had higher Injury Severity Scores. Independent risk factors for VTE included thoracic injuries [odds ratio (OR): 6.9; 95% confidence interval (CI): 1.4–35.1] and spinal injuries (OR: 37.4; 95% CI: 3.5–396.7). The greatest risk of VTE was in children with central venous catheters (OR: 64.0; 95% CI: 16.8–243.9). ***Conclusion:*** Older children with high Injury Severity Scores, thoracic injuries, spinal injuries or venous catheters are at risk for VTE. Because VTE prophylaxis, screening and treatment are associated with complications and costs, it is essential to identify subgroups of pediatric patients in whom these strategies might be studied.

Introduction

Venous thromboembolism [VTE; deep vein thrombosis (DVT) and pulmonary embolism] is a common disease [1–3]. Generally, the incidence of VTE is considered to be lower in children than in adults. As much as 30% of adults admitted to critical care units are reported to have DVT when screened [2]. In children, studies described a low incidence ranging from 0.05 to 0.1% in hospitalized children with risk factors [1, 4–6].

In adults, surgery and trauma are considered to be independent risk factors for VTE [3, 5]. Recently, two studies [1, 6] reported a low incidence of VTE in injured children admitted to the hospital, but many of the patients were not seriously injured, and most were hospitalized in nontrauma centers. Thus, information on risk factors and on the incidence of VTE is scarce for severely injured children [1, 6]. A number of factors have been reported to increase the risk of VTE after injury including spinal fractures and spinal cord injury. Factors that have been suspected to increase the risk include long bone fractures, pelvic fractures and head injuries [7]. Because VTE pro-

KARGER

Fax +41 61 306 12 34
E-Mail karger@karger.ch
www.karger.com

0001–5792/06/1154–0198$23.50/0

Accessible online at:
www.karger.com/aha

Claude Cyr
Faculté de Médecine, Université de Sherbrooke
3001, 12ème Avenue Nord, Sherbrooke, J1H 5N4 (Canada)
Tel. +1 819 346 1110, ext. 14634, Fax +1 819 564 5398
E-Mail claude.cyr@usherbrooke.ca

phylaxis is associated with complications, it is essential to identify subgroups of trauma patients in whom the benefit of prophylaxis will outweigh the risk.

The aim of our study was to determine the incidence of VTE and risk factors in severely injured children.

Methods

After institutional review board approval, we conducted a study in two trauma centers. We used the hospital-based trauma registries to identify a cohort of severely injured children (age <18 years; admitted in a pediatric intensive care unit or length of stay >72 h).

Subjects

Children with any International Classification of Diseases, Ninth Revision (ICD-9) discharge diagnosis ranging from 800 to 959, excluding late effects of injuries (905–909), foreign bodies (930–939), and burns (940–949) were considered to be trauma victims. We limited the analysis to patients with a principal diagnosis of trauma, that is those patients in whom the first diagnosis field was a trauma-related diagnosis, as defined above. This approach reduced the possibility of miscoding patients with iatrogenic injuries as trauma patients [1, 8].

Venous Thromboembolic Disease

Subjects with any ICD-9 discharge diagnoses of phlebitis or thrombophlebitis of the deep veins of the lower extremities, iliac vein, inferior vena cava, or other, unspecified veins or sites (451.1, 451.11, 451.19, 451.2, 451.81, 453.2, 451.2, 453.8, and 453.9) or those with involvement of the deep veins of the upper extremities (451.83, 451.89, and 451.84) were considered to have DVT. Subjects with any diagnoses of pulmonary embolus and infarction (415.1, 415.19, and 415.11) were classified as such. For the purposes of this analysis, venous thromboembolic disease refers to either DVT or pulmonary embolus as defined above [8].

Risk Factors for Venous Thromboembolic Disease

Several potential risk factors for venous thromboembolic disease were considered and abstracted from the registries. Age groups (0–4, 5–9, 10–14 and 15–18 years) along with several specific diagnoses and procedures were identified and categorized by ICD-9 diagnoses or procedure codes. These included pelvic fractures, spinal cord injuries and major vascular injuries involving the chest, abdomen, and extremities exclusive of the pulmonary vasculature, splanchnic, and renal vessels. We also considered head, chest, abdominal, spine, and extremity injuries to be potential risk factors.

The Injury Severity Score, a global measure of anatomic injury severity, was calculated by summing the squares of the highest abbreviated injury scale (AIS) scores from the three different body regions with the highest abbreviated injury scale scores [9, 10].

A variety of procedures were considered to potentially increase the risk of VTE, including craniotomy or craniectomy, laparotomy, central venous catheterization, operations on the spine, or operative reduction and internal fixation of bone fractures. These procedures were identified by ICD-9 procedure codes.

Statistical Analysis

Rates were calculated per 1,000 admissions. All risk factors with statistically significant ($p < 0.05$) association with VTE were entered in a logistic regression model to determine the independent association of these variables with VTE.

Results

There were 3,291 pediatric trauma-related admissions in the two institutions that fulfilled the definition for severe trauma. Eleven patients had a discharge diagnosis of VTE, resulting in a rate of 3.3/1,000 admissions. Of these 11 patients, 8 had isolated DVT, 3 had isolated pulmonary emboli, and no patient had a diagnosis of both DVT and pulmonary embolism. Overall, patients with VTE were older (mean age: 11.9 vs. 8.5 years; p = 0.03; Student's t test). The risk of VTE increased with age. Patients in the 15- to 18-year age group had an odds ratio (OR) of 19.5 [95% confidence interval (CI), 1.1–361.9] compared to the 0- to 5-year age group. There were no deaths associated with VTE in our cohort.

VTE was associated with severe injuries (Injury Severity Score ≥9; OR: 5.3; 95% CI: 1.6–17.3). When specific injuries were considered, patients with spinal injuries were more likely to be affected (OR: 23.4; 95% CI: 3.2–170.8). Thoracic and abdominal injuries were associated with VTE (OR: 13.8, 95% CI: 3.7–51.2, and OR: 7.7, 95% CI: 2.3–26.2, respectively).

Procedures that were associated with an increased risk of VTE included operations on the spine (OR: 54.8; 95% CI: 8.2–363.6), laparotomy (OR: 29.8; 95% CI: 4.2–213.5) and central venous catheters (OR: 4.8; 95% CI: 1.5–15.8).

Multivariate Analysis

In our logistic regression model, Injury Severity Score, increasing age, chest injuries (OR: 6.9; 95% CI: 1.4–35.1), spine injury (OR: 37.4; 95% CI: 3.5–396.7) and central venous catheters (OR: 64.0; 95% CI: 16.8–243.9) were independently associated with VTE.

Discussion

A number of factors have been reported to increase the risk of VTE in children. The results of our analysis indicate that the rate of VTE after severe pediatric trauma is approximately 0.3%. The risk of VTE was not uniform across age groups. The rate of VTE in the present study is small but slightly higher than reported in other studies of injured children ranging from 0.07 to 0.77 per 1,000 discharges [1, 6]. However, it is similar to the rate associated with subgroups of severely injured children [1]. The rate is likely understated but the prevalence of VTE in severely injured children appears to be significantly lower than that in adults.

Older children with higher Injury Severity Scores, thoracic injuries, spinal injuries or central venous catheters are at risk for VTE. We did not confirm the association between head injury and VTE [1]. The existing evidence supports the presence of two risk factors of VTE in adult patients: spinal fractures and spinal cord injuries [7]. Impaired venous return from the lower extremities and abnormal coagulation factors are thought to predispose patients with spinal cord injuries to VTE [11–13].

The independent association between Injury Severity Score and VTE risk in pediatric trauma is consistent with reports of an increased risk of VTE in adults with major trauma [3, 7, 12]. The associated risk factors for the development of VTE identified in this study are similar to what is reported in adult trauma [3, 12–14]. There were no deaths associated with VTE in this cohort. The Canadian Thrombophilia Registry reported a mortality rate of 2.2% directly attributed to VTE; all children who died had central venous catheter-associated thrombosis [5].

This study has some limitations. It is based only on clinically significant VTE, which is known to be much less common than VTE diagnosed with active screening [1, 15, 16]. Although there is little dispute regarding the value of testing symptomatic patients for DVT, the overall accuracy of screening ultrasound in the asymptomatic patient is less clear. Prior reports on the prevalence of VTE in adults usually were based on data from trauma centers where patients underwent routine screening for VTE. To our knowledge, there is no data on the prevalence of VTE on the basis of active screening in injured children. Our approach is useful in defining high-risk groups that warrant particular attention and may be candidate for thromboprophylaxis. However, the effect of preexisting, permanent risk factors on the incidence of thromboembolism in injured children is largely unknown. Common primary thrombophilias, such as the factor V Leiden and prothrombin 20210A mutations, have not been evaluated in this population.

In conclusion, this study identifies the prevalence and specific risk factors for the development of VTE in severely injured children. Older children with thoracic injuries, spinal injuries and/or the presence of a central venous catheter are at higher risk for VTE. This population may benefit from routine prophylaxis and/or screening. Prospective and adequately sized studies should be done to quantify risk and evaluate specific prevention strategies.

References

1 Vavilala MS, Nathens AB, Jurkovich GJ, Mackenzie E, Rivara FP: Risk factors for venous thromboembolism in pediatric trauma. J Trauma 2002;52:922–927.

2 Attia J, Ray JG, Cook DJ, Douketis J, Ginsberg JS, Geerts WH: Deep vein thrombosis and its prevention in critically ill adults. Arch Intern Med 2001;161:1268–1279.

3 Heit JA, Silverstein MD, Mohr DN, Petterson TM, O'Fallon WM, Melton LJ 3rd: Risk factors for deep vein thrombosis and pulmonary embolism: a population-based case-control study. Arch Intern Med 2000;160:809–815.

4 Rohrer M, Cutler B, MacDougall E, Herrmann JB, Anderson FA Jr, Wheeler HB: A prospective study of the incidence of deep venous thrombosis in hospitalized children. J Vasc Surg 1996;24:46–49.

5 Anderson FA, Spencer FA: Risk factors for venous thromboembolism. Circulation 2003; 107:I-9–I-16.

6 Grandas O, Klar M, Goldman M, Filston H: Deep venous thrombosis in the pediatric trauma population: an unusual event-report of three cases. Am Surg 2000;66:273–276.

7 Rogers FB, Cipolle MD, Velmahos G, Rozycki G, Luchette FA: Practice Management Guidelines for the Prevention of Venous Thromboembolism in Trauma Patients: the EAST Practice Management Guidelines Work Group. J Trauma 2002;53:142–164.

8 MacKenzie EJ, Steinwachs DM, Shankar B: Classifying trauma severity based on hospital discharge diagnoses: validation of an ICD-9CM to AIS-85 conversion table. Med Care 1989;27:412–422.

9 Association for the Advancement of Automotive Medicine. The Abbreviated Injury Scale, 1990 Revision. Des Plaines, Association for the Advancement of Automotive Medicine, 1990.

10 Baker SP, O'Neill B, Haddon W Jr, Long WB: The injury severity score: a method for describing patients with multiple injuries and evaluating emergency care. J Trauma 1974;14:187–196.

11 Merli G, Crabbe S, Paluzzi R, Fritz D: Etiology, incidence, and prevention of deep vein thrombosis in acute spinal cord injury. Arch Phys Med Rehabil 1993;74:1199–1205.

12 Geerts W, Code K, Jay R, Chen E, Szalai J: A prospective study of venous thromboembolism after major trauma. N Engl J Med 1994; 331:1601–1606.

13 Napolitano L, Garlapati V, Heard S, Silva W, Cutler B, O'Neil A, Anderson FA Jr, Wheeler H: Asymptomatic deep venous thrombosis in the trauma patient: is an aggressive screening protocol justified? J Trauma 1995;39:651–659.

14 Andrew M, David M, Adams M, Ali K, Anderson R, Barnard D, Bernstein M, Brisson L, Cairney B, DeSai D, Israels S, Jardine L, Luke B, Massicotte P, Silva M: Venous thromboembolic complications (VTE) in children: first analyses of the Canadian Registry of VTE. Blood 1994;83:1251–1257.

15 Knudson MM, Collins JA, Goodman SB, McCrory DW: Thromboembolism following multiple trauma. J Trauma 1992;32:2–11.

16 Knudson MM, Lewis FR, Clinton A, Atkinson K, Megerman J: Prevention of venous thromboembolism in trauma patients. J Trauma 1994;37:480–487.

Acta Hæmatologica

Acta Haematol 2006;115:201–206
DOI: 10.1159/000090936

Central Venous Line-Related Thrombosis in Children

Shoshana Revel-Vilk

Pediatric Hematology/Oncology Unit, Hadassah Hebrew University Medical Center, Jerusalem, Israel

Key Words
Central venous lines · Children · Risk factors · Prophylaxis

Abstract
Central venous lines are used in critically ill children and in children with chronic conditions for the administration of intravenous therapy, such as fluids, medications, total parenteral nutrition and blood products. Although the use of central venous lines has greatly improved the quality of care in these children, these catheters may cause serious mechanical, infectious and thrombotic complications. The reported frequency of catheter thrombosis in children is low as 5% in studies including only symptomatic cases and high as 50% in studies where patients are systematically screened for catheter-related thrombosis. The risk factors for catheter-related thrombosis in children are associated with the methods used for catheter insertion and with individual patient characteristics, underlying diagnosis and treatment. The management of catheter-related thrombosis is largely dependent on the requirement of the catheter. If no longer required or nonfunctioning the catheter should be removed. If access is still required and the catheter is functioning, treatment with anticoagulation is recommended in the absence of contraindications. The management of radiographically detected asymptomatic thrombosis in children is less clear. Clinical studies of prophylaxis for catheter-related thrombosis are inconclusive and no definitive recommendations for prophylaxis in adults or in children with central venous thrombosis can be made. Properly designed studies are needed to assess the role of prophylactic anticoagulation for preventing catheter-related thrombosis.

Central venous lines (CVL) are used in children for administration of intravenous therapy, such as fluids, medications, total parenteral nutrition (TPN), and blood products. The majority of children requiring CVL are children with cancer, children requiring long-term TPN, and children admitted to intensive care units. Central lines in children are usually placed into the upper venous system through peripheral veins from the arm or through major vessels such as the subclavian and jugular veins. The two mostly used CVLs in children are tunneled central venous catheters (single or double lumen) and implantable central venous access ports.

The use of CVLs is associated with mechanical, infectious and thrombotic complications. Thrombotic complications are thought to arise by several mechanisms: damage to the vessel wall by the catheter or by substances

KARGER

Fax +41 61 306 12 34
E-Mail karger@karger.ch
www.karger.com

0001–5792/06/1154–0201$23.50/0

Accessible online at:
www.karger.com/aha

Shoshana Revel-Vilk
Pediatric Hematology/Oncology Unit
Hadassah Hebrew University Hospital, POB 12000
IL–91200 Jerusalem (Israel)
Tel. +972 2 677 7408, Fax +972 2 677 7833, E-Mail shoshanav@hadassah.org.il

infused through the catheter, such as TPN, and chemotherapy, disrupted blood flow, and thrombogenic catheter materials. Three types of CVL-related thrombosis may develop: sleeve thrombus, intraluminal thrombus and mural thrombus. A sleeve thrombus can occlude the catheter tip creating a valve effect. This thrombus may be a source for microbial colonization and may rarely detach and cause pulmonary embolism. An intraluminal thrombus can cause blockage or catheter dysfunction requiring local instillation of thrombolytic agents. Mural thrombosis can totally or partially occlude the vessel lumen and cause localized symptoms, such as arm swelling, shoulder pain, neck swelling, headache and development of the superior vena cava syndrome. However, the gradual development of a mural thrombosis and the development of venous collaterals may result in asymptomatic occurrence of deep vein thrombosis. Dysfunctional CVL, difficulty in obtaining blood return or increased resistance during infusion may be the first and only signs of the development of a fibrin sheath or mural thrombosis of the upper venous system.

The potential serious complications of CVL-related thrombosis include repeat anesthesia for CVL placement, loss of subsequent intravenous access, recurrent thrombosis, pulmonary embolism, postthrombotic syndrome and death. In the Canadian registry the mortality, recurrent thrombosis and postthrombotic syndrome from CVL-related thrombosis were 3.7, 6.5 and 9.5%, respectively [1]. Theoretically, even asymptomatic CVL-related thrombosis diagnosed during radiographic imaging performed for other reasons or diagnosed secondary to loss of CVL patency may have similar rates of complications [2]. Although the benefits from using CVLs in children outweigh the potential risks from CVLs, better understanding of the risks factors for development of thrombosis and improved prophylaxis and treatment of CVL-related thrombosis may further decrease the rate of complications and augment the benefit of CVL in children.

Frequency of CVL-Related Thrombosis

The reported prevalence of CVL-related thrombosis in children varies, reflecting different underlying diagnoses, treatment protocols, diagnostic tests and index of suspicion. In the Canadian registry the incidence of CVL-related thrombosis in children with different diseases was 3.5 per 100,000 hospital admissions [1]. In children with acute lymphoblastic leukemia (ALL) treated with *L*-asparaginase and steroids the reported prevalence of symptomatic thrombosis was 5–11% [3, 4], while the prevalence of asymptomatic thrombosis (diagnosed with routine bilateral venography, magnetic resonance imaging, ultrasound and echocardiography) was 37.5% [3]. The prevalence of symptomatic thrombosis in children with other types of cancer (non-ALL) was 2–6% [5, 6]. Studies that systematically screened children with cancer and CVL for thrombosis found a variable prevalence depending on the screening tool. Routine echocardiography in 156 children with cancer found a prevalence of 8.8% of right atrial thrombosis [7]. Spiral computed tomography in 25 children with cancer whose CVL had been removed at least 2 months previously found a prevalence of 12% of CVL-related thrombosis [8]. Screening with Doppler ultrasound in 41 children with a Hickman catheter found a prevalence of 44% of CVL-related thrombosis [9]. Screening with contrast venography in 24 children with subcutaneous ports found a prevalence of 50% of CVL-related thrombosis [10]. Most of these episodes were clinically silent. In the PARKAA study (Prophylactic Antithrombin Replacement in Kids with ALL Treated with Asparaginase), ultrasound was demonstrated to be insensitive compared to venography for CVL-related intrathoracic thrombosis, but more sensitive for jugular vein thrombosis [11], suggesting that a combination of ultrasound and venograpy imaging is required for accurate diagnosis of CVL-related thrombosis in the upper venous system [12]. In the future, magnetic resonance imaging may become a noninvasive alternative for invasive venography for the detection of CVL-related thrombosis [13, 14].

In children receiving home TPN, the incidence of CVL-related thrombosis was reported to range from 1 to 80%, with the lowest frequencies reflecting the clinical diagnosis of thrombosis and the highest frequencies reflecting venographic evidence of thrombosis [15]. In children with short-term catheter placement in an intensive care unit, the incidence of symptomatic CVL-related thrombosis was 3% [16], while the prevalence with ultrasound screening was reported as 18 and 35%, in two separate studies [17, 18]. In children with hemophilia, contrast venography identified CVL-related thrombosis in 8/15 and 13/16 children, of whom only 4/15 and 3/16 had clinical signs of thrombosis [19, 20]. The prevalence of symptomatic CVL-related thrombosis in patients with cystic fibrosis was reported to be 5–17% [21, 22]. In patients with sickle cell disease and thalassemia, the reported prevalence of CVL-related thrombosis was 33 and 35%, respectively [23, 24]. The prevalence of CVL-related thrombosis in children with dysfunctional venous catheter was not systematically studied. Although some studies suggested that loss of CVL patency is predictive for occurrence of CVL-related thrombosis [25], other published results in this area are conflicting. Knowing the actual risk for the development of CVL-related thrombosis is important for the calculation of the benefit/risk ratio in the various patient populations.

Risk Factors

The various risk factors suggested for CVL-related thrombosis can be categorized into those related to the catheter, those related to the individual and those related to the underlying disease and its treatment. In adults with cancer and CVL the following risk factors were reported: type of CVL (tunneled vs. totally implanted), type of infusion (clear fluid vs. TPN), platelet count at the time of catheter placement, size of catheter (single vs. double lumen) and position of catheter [26]. In children with ALL insertion of the CVL to the left side, to the subclavian vein and percutaneous insertion of CVL were associated with an increased incidence of thrombosis [27]. No association was found between platelet count and the occurrence of thrombosis. In children with various types of cancer both infectious and mechanical complications were significantly more common among surgically placed CVLs than those placed radiologically [5]. The contribution of inherited and acquired thrombophilia to CVL-related thrombosis is controversial. While some studies in children with CVL-related thrombosis showed a very high prevalence of thrombophilia [4, 28], other groups that followed children or adults with CVL-related thrombosis found a low prevalence of thrombophilic markers [9, 27, 29, 30]. In children with cancer, the treatment regimens and inherited thrombophilia defects rather than inherited thrombophilia alone were found to be important in the pathogenesis of symptomatic VTE [6, 31, 32]. In children with hemophilia the occurrence of CVL-related thrombosis was related to the duration of catheter placement, with no patient whose CVL was in place fewer than 48 months having an abnormal venogram [19]. An association between the infusion of high doses of factor VIII, as part of an immune tolerance protocol, and the development of thrombosis was also suggested [33]. In children with short-term catheter use treated in an intensive care unit, the rate of thrombosis was higher for femoral access, long-indwelling catheters, presence of cancer and young age [16, 18]. The hypercoagulability in sickle cell disease and in thalassemia could explain the increased risk for CVL-related thrombosis [34, 35]. Recognition of the risk factors for CVL-related complications may potentially reduce the rate of complications and prolong the use of these essential devices.

Prophylaxis

The potential complications of CVL-related thrombosis led to development of clinical studies of prophylaxis [36]. Bern et al. [37] reported the efficacy of daily low-dose warfarin (1 mg) in prevention of CVL-related thrombosis in cancer patients with subcutaneous ports. A subsequent study in cancer patients with tunneled Hickman catheters found no benefit for the routine use of low-dose warfarin for prevention of symptomatic CVL-related thrombosis [38]. Whether the contradictory conclusion is related to differences in patient population, type of catheter or time of starting warfarin prophylaxis is unclear (table 1). The efficacy of low-molecular-weight heparin in CVL prophylaxis was also studied in randomized studies (table 1). In adults, the use of low-molecular-weight heparin was safe and effective in prevention of asymptomatic CVL-related thrombosis [39]. In children, the use of low-molecular-weight heparin for prevention of CVL-related thrombosis was safe, but its efficacy was unclear due to small sample size [40]. A study comparing low-dose warfarin and low-molecular-weight heparin for CVL prophylaxis showed comparable benefit-risk ratios [41]. Cohort studies following cancer patients receiving low-dose warfarin [29, 42, 43] or low-molecular-weight heparin [44–46] for CVL prophylaxis have shown different rates of efficacy (table 2). In one of those studies, it was suggested that higher doses of unfractionated heparin flushing (>500 U/ml) could reduce the rate of CVL-related thrombosis [46]. Similarly, in a meta-analysis prophylactic unfractionated heparin reduced CVL-related VTE (RR: 0.43, 95% confidence interval: 0.23–0.78) [47]. Heparin-bonded CVLs were also shown to reduce the risk for thrombosis [48–50]. The role of adding urokinase to the heparin flushing in the prevention of CVL-related thrombosis is unclear [51–54]. Thus, available studies do not allow definitive recommendations for CVL prophylaxis in adults or in children and properly designed studies are needed to assess the role of prophylactic anticoagulation, the recommended dosage and frequency of unfractionated heparin instillation in CVL and the use of urokinase and/or heparin-bonded CVLs for preventing CVL-related thrombosis.

Table 1. Prospective randomized studies of CVL prophylaxis

Study	Population	CVL type	Intervention	Thrombotic events	
				symptomatic	symptomatic + asymptomatic
Bern et al. [37]	all cancer, adults	ports	1 mg warfarin, 3 days before insertion	4/42 (9.5)	4/42 (9.5)
			no warfarin	10/40 (25)	15/40 (37.5)
Monreal et al. [39]	all cancer, adults	ports	2,500 U fragmin	–	1/16 (6.3)
			no fragmin	–	8/13 (61.5)
Heaton et al. [38]	hematology malignancy, adults	Hickman	1 mg warfarin, day of insertion	2/51 (3.9)	–
			no warfarin	1/51 (2)	–
Mismetti et al. [41]	solid tumors, adults	ports	1 mg warfarin, 3 days before insertion	2/24 (8.3)	4/24 (16.7)
			2,850 U nadroparin, day of insertion	1/21 (4.8)	6/21 (28.6)
Massicotte et al. [40]	different diagnoses, children	Hickman, ports	30–50 U/kg reviparin sodium	3/77 (3.9)	11/77 (14.1)
			no reviparin sodium	3/80 (3.8)	10/80 (12.5)

Figures in parentheses represent percentage.

Table 2. Cohort studies of CVL prophylaxis

Study	Population	CVL type	Intervention	Symptomatic thrombosis
Nightingale et al. [42]	GI malignancy, adults	Hickman	1 mg warfarin, day of insertion	42/949 (4.4)
Boraks et al. [43]	hematology malignancy, adults	Hickman	1 mg warfarin, day of insertion	5/108 (4.6)
Ratcliffe et al. [29]	solid tumors, adults	Hickman	1 mg warfarin, day of insertion	7/55 (12.7)
Largo et al. [44]	bone marrow transplant, adults	Hickman	no prophylaxis	10/163 (6.1)
			2,850 U nadroparin, day of insertion	10/123 (8.1)
			5,700 U nadroparin, day of insertion	7/102 (6.7)
Elhasid et al. [45]	leukemia, children		0.45–1.33 mg/kg enoxaparin, 1st dose of *L*-asparaginase	0/41
Lersch et al. [46]	all cancer, adults	ports	2,500 U dalteparin, day of insertion	7/119 (5.9)
			5,000 U dalteparin, day of insertion	2/54 (3.7)

Figures in parentheses represent percentage. GI = Gastrointestinal.

Treatment

The recommended management of acute and symptomatic CVL-related thrombosis is clear and largely depends on the requirement for the CVL. If the CVL is no longer required, or is nonfunctioning, it should be removed [55]. Anticoagulation therapy 3–5 days prior to CVL removal is recommended. If CVL access is still required and is functioning, the CVL may be left in place, and anticoagulation therapy should be given according to previously published recommendations [55]. After completion of the first 3 months of anticoagulant therapy, switching to prophylaxis doses of anticoagulation therapy is recommended until the CVL is removed [55].

The recommended management of radiographically detected asymptomatic CVL-related thrombosis is less clear. If the CVL is no longer required, it should be removed. If CVL access is still required, the recommended management is based mainly on expert opinion and less on evidence-based data. Thus, as in children asymptomatic CVL-related thrombosis is believed to have clinical importance, treatment with anticoagulation is recommended in the absence of contraindications [2]. However, in such circumstances, the need for full dose anticoagulation is not clear [56].

References

1 Massicotte MP, Dix D, Monagle P, Adams M, Andrew M: Central venous catheter related thrombosis in children: analysis of the Canadian registry of venous thromboembolic complications. J Pediatr 1998;133:770–776.

2 Chan AK, Deveber G, Monagle P, Brookers LA, Massicottes MP: Venous thrombosis in children. J Thromb Haemost 2003;1:1443–1455.

3 Mitchell LG, Andrew M, Hanna K, Abshire T, Halton J, Anderson R, Cherrick I, Desai S, Mahoney D, McCuster P, Wu J, Dahl G, Chait P, de Veber G, Lee KJ, Mikulis D, Ginsberg J, Way C; Prophylactic Antithrombin Replacement in Kids with Acute Lymphoblastic Leukemia Treated with Asparaginase Group (PARKAA): A prospective cohort study determining the prevalence of thrombotic events in children with acute lymphoblastic leukemia and a central venous line who are treated with *L*-asparaginase: results of the Prophylactic Antithrombin Replacement in Kids with Acute Lymphoblastic Leukemia Treated with Asparaginase (PARKAA) Study. Cancer 2003;97: 508–516.

4 Nowak-Gottl U, Wermes C, Junker R, Koch HG, Schobess R, Fleischhack G, Schwabe D, Ehrenforth S: Prospective evaluation of the thrombotic risk in children with acute lymphoblastic leukemia carrying the MTHFR TT 677 genotype, the prothrombin G20210A variant, and further prothrombotic risk factors. Blood 1999;93:1595–1599.

5 Basford TJ, Poenaru D, Silva M: Comparison of delayed complications of central venous catheters placed surgically or radiologically in pediatric oncology patients. J Pediatr Surg 2003;5:788–792.

6 Wermes C, von Depka Prondzinski M, Lichtinghagen R, Barthels M, Welte K, Sykora KW: Clinical relevance of genetic risk factors for thrombosis in paediatric oncology patients with central venous catheters. Eur J Pediatr 1999;158(suppl 3):S143–S146.

7 Korones DN, Buzzard CJ, Asselin BL, Harris JP: Right atrial thrombi in children with cancer and indwelling catheters. J Pediatr 1996; 128:841–846.

8 Wiliams JA, Hidson M, Rao B, Luo X, Lott L, Kaste SC: Late vascular occlusion of central lines in pediatrics malignancy. Pediatrics 1998;101:E7.

9 Ruud E, Holmstrom H, Natvig S, Wesenberg F: Prevalence of thrombophilia and central venous catheter-associated neck vein thrombosis in children with cancer – a prospective study. Med Pediatr Oncol 2002;38:405–410.

10 Glaser DW, Medeiros D, Rollins N, Buchanan GR: Catheter-related thrombosis in children with cancer. J Pediatr 2001;138:255–259.

11 Male C, Chait P, Ginsberg JS, Hanna K, Andrew M, Halton J, Anderson R, McCusker P, Wu J, Abshire T, Cherrick I, Mahoney D, Mitchell L: Comparison of venography and ultrasound for the diagnosis of asymptomatic deep vein thrombosis in the upper body in children: results of the PARKAA study. Prophylactic Antithrombin Replacement in Kids with ALL Treated with Asparaginase. Thromb Haemost 2002;87:593–598.

12 Male C, Kuhle S, Mitchell L: Diagnosis of venous thromboembolism in children. Semin Thromb Hemost 2003;29:377–390.

13 Kaste SC, Gronemeyer SA, Hoffer FA, Mandrell BN, Wilimas JA: Pilot study of noninvasive detection of venous occlusions from central venous access devices in children treated for acute lymphoblastic leukemia. Pediatr Radiol 1999;29:570–574.

14 Shankar KR, Abernethy LJ, Das KSV, Roche CJ, Pizer BL, Lioyd DA, Losty PD: Magnetic resonance venography in assessing venous patency after multiple venous catheters. J Pediatr Surg 2002;37:175–179.

15 Andrew M, Marzinotto V, Pencharz P, Zlotkin S, Burrows P, Ingram J, Adams M, Filler R: A cross-sectional study of catheter-related thrombosis in children receiving total parenteral nutrition at home. J Pediatr 1995;126:358–363.

16 Casado-Flores J, Barja J, Martino R, Serrano A, Valdivielso A: Complications of central venous catheterization in critically ill children. Pediatr Crit Care Med 2001;2:57–62.

17 Talbott GA, Winters WD, Bratton SL, O'Rourke PP: A prospective study of femoral catheter-related thrombosis in children. Arch Pediatr Adolesc Med 1995;149:288–291.

18 Beck C, Dubois J, Grignon A, Lacroix J, David M: Incidence and risk factors of catheter related deep vein thrombosis in a pediatric intensive care unit: a prospective study. J Pediatr 1998;133:237–241.

19 Journeycake JM, Quinn CT, Miller KL, Zajac JL, Buchanan GR: Catheter-related deep venous thrombosis in children with hemophilia. Blood 2001;98:1727–1731.

20 Price VE, Carcao M, Connolly B, Daneman A, Temple M, Stain AM, Sung L, Al-Tralbosi H, Blanchette VS: A prospective, longitudinal study of central venous catheter-related deep vein thrombosis in boys with hemophilia. J Thromb Haemost 2004;2:737–742.

21 Munck A, Malbezin S, Bloch J, Gerardin M, Lebourgeois M, Derelle J, Bremont F, Sermet I, Munck MR, Navarro J: Follow-up of 452 totally implantable vascular devices in cystic fibrosis patients. Eur Respir J 2004;23:430–434.

22 Aitken ML, Tonelli MR: Complications of indwelling catheters in cystic fibrosis: a 10-year review. Chest 2000;118:1598–1602.

23 Jeng MR, Feusner J, Skibola C, Vichinsky E: Central venous catheter complications in sickle cell disease. Am J Hematol 2002;69:103–108.

24 Finkelstein Y, Yaniv I, Berant M, Zilber R, Garty B, Epstein O, Lahav Y, Tamary H: Central venous line thrombosis in children and young adults with thalassemia major. Pediatr Hematol Oncol 2004;21:375–381.

25 Andrew M, Monagle P, Brooker LA: Epidemiology of venous thromboembolism events; in Andrew M, Monagle P, Brooker L (eds): Thromboembolic Complications during Infancy and Childhood. Hamilton, Decker, 2000, pp 111–146.

26 Monreal M, Davant E: Thrombotic complications of central venous catheters in cancer patients. Acta Haematol 2001;106:69–72.

27 Male C, Chait P, Andrew M, Hanna K, Julian J, Mitchell L: Central venous line-related thrombosis in children: association with central venous line location and insertion technique. Blood 2003;101:4273–4278.

28 Nowak-Gottl U, Dubbers A, Kececioglu D, Koch HG, Kotthoff S, Runde J, Vielhaber H: Factor V Leiden, protein C, and lipoprotein (a) in catheter-related thrombosis in childhood: a prospective study. J Pediatr 1997;131:608–612.

29 Ratcliffe M, Broadfoot C, Davidson M, Kelly KF, Greaves M: Thrombosis, markers of thrombotic risk, indwelling central venous catheter and antithrombotic prophylaxis using low-dose warfarin in subjects with malignant disease. Clin Lab Haematol 1999;21:353–357.

30 Revel-Vilk S, Chan A, Bauman M, Massicotte P: Incidence of congenital prothrombotic disorders in an unselected cohort of children with venous thromboembolic disease. J Thromb Haemost 2003;1:915–921.

31 Mauz-Korholz C, Junker R, Gobel U, Nowak-Gottl U: Prothrombotic risk factors in children with acute lymphoblastic leukemia treated with delayed *E. coli* asparaginase (COALL-92 and 97 protocols). Thromb Haemost 2000;83: 840–843.

32 Athale UA, Chan AKC: Thrombosis in children with acute lymphoblastic leukemia. Part III. Pathogenesis of thrombosis in children with acute lymphoblastic leukemia: effects of host environment. Thromb Res 2003;111: 321–327.

33 Carcao MD, Connolly BL, Chait P, Stain AM, Acebes M, Massicotte P, Blanchette VS: Central venous catheter-related thrombosis presenting as superior vena cava syndrome in a haemophilic patient with inhibitors. Haemophilia 2003;9:578–583.

34 Ataga KI, Orringer EP: Hypercoagulability in sickle cell disease: a curious paradox. Am J Med 2003;15:721–728.

35 Eldor A, Rachmilewitz EA: The hypercoagulable state in thalassemia. Blood 2002;99:36–43.

36 Klerk CPW, Smorenburg SM, Buller HR: Thrombosis prophylaxis in patient populations with a central venous catheter. Arch Intern Med 2003;163:1913–1921.
37 Bern MM, Lokich JJ, Wallach SR, Bothe A, Benotti PN, Arkin DF, et al: Very low doses of warfarin can prevent thrombosis in central venous catheters. A randomized prospective trial. Ann Intern Med 1990;112:423–428.
38 Heaton DC, Han DY, Inder A: Minidose (1 mg) warfarin as prophylaxis for central vein catheter thrombosis. Intern Med J 2002;32: 84–88.
39 Monreal M, Alastrue A, Rull M, Mira X, Muxart J, Rosell R, Abad A: Upper extremity deep venous thrombosis in cancer patients with venous access devices – prophylaxis with a low molecular weight heparin (Fragmin). Thromb Haemost 1996;75:251–253.
40 Massicotte P, Julian JA, Gent M, Shields K, Marzinotto V, Szechtman B, Chan AC, Andrew M; PROTEKT Study Group: An open-label randomized controlled trial of low molecular weight heparin for the prevention of central venous line-related thrombotic complications in children: the PROTEKT trial. Thromb Res 2003;109:101–108.
41 Mismetti P, Mille D, Laporte S, Charlet V, Buchmuller-Cordier A, Jacquin JP, Fournel P, Dutrey-Dupagne C, Decousus H: Low-molecular-weight heparin (nadroparin) and very low doses of warfarin in the prevention of upper extremity thrombosis in cancer patients with indwelling long-term central venous catheters: a pilot randomized trial. Haematologica 2003; 88:67–73.
42 Nightingale CE, Norman A, Cunningham D, Young J, Webb A, Filshie J: A prospective analysis of 949 long-term central venous access catheters for ambulatory chemotherapy in patients with gastrointestinal malignancy. Eur J Cancer 1997;33:398–403.
43 Boraks P, Seale J, Price J, Bass G, Ethell M, Keeling D, Mahendra P, Baglin T, Marcus R: Prevention of central venous catheter associated thrombosis using minidose warfarin in patients with haematological malignancies. Br J Haematol 1998;101:483–486.
44 Largo SW, Verdonck LF, Borel Rinkes IHM, Dekker AW: No effect of nadroparin prophylaxis in the prevention of central venous catheter (CVC)-associated thrombosis in bone marrow transplant recipients. Bone Marrow Transplant 2000;26:1103–1106.
45 Elhasid R, Lanir N, Sharon R, Weyl Ben Arush M, Levin C: Prophylactic therapy with enoxaparin during *L*-asparaginase treatment in children with acute lymphoblastic leukemia. Blood Coagul Fibrinolysis 2001;12:367–370.
46 Lersch C, Kotowa W, Fung S, Janssen D: Prophylaxis of port system-associated thromboses in advanced oncology patients using heparin flushing. J Cancer Res Clin Oncol 2004;130: 235–241.
47 Randolph AG, Cook DJ, Gonzales CA, Andrew M: Benefit of heparin in central venous and pulmonary artery catheters. Chest 1998; 113:165–171.
48 Efsing HO, Lindblad B, Mark J, Wolff T: Thromboembolic complications from central venous catheters: a comparison of three catheter materials. World J Surg 1983;7:419–423.
49 Krafte-Jacobs B, Sivit CJ, Mejia R, Pollack MM: Catheter-related thrombosis in critically ill children: comparison of catheters with and without heparin bonding. J Pediatr 1995;126: 50–54.
50 Pierce CM, Wade A, Mok Q: Heparin-bonded central venous lines reduce thrombotic and infective complications in critically ill children. Intensive Care Med 2000;26:967–972.
51 Ray CE Jr, Shenoy SS, McCarthy PL, Broderick KA, Kaufman JA: Weekly prophylaxis urokinase instillation in tunneled central venous access devices. J Vasc Interv Radiol 1999;10: 1330–1334.
52 Solomon B, Moore J, Arthur C, Prince HM: Lack of efficacy of twice-weekly urokinase in the prevention of complications associated with Hickman catheters: a multicenter randomized comparison of urokinase versus heparin. Eur J Cancer 2001;37:2379–2384.
53 Kalmanti M, Germanakis J, Stiakaki E, Syfridaki C, Christidou A, Tsetis D, Vardas P: Prophylaxis with urokinase in pediatric oncology patients with central venous catheters. Pediatr Hematol Oncol 2002;19:173–179.
54 Dillon PW, Jones GR, Bagnall-Reeb HA, Buckely JD, Weiner ES, Haase GM, Children's Oncology Group: Prophylactic urokinase in the management of long-term venous access devices in children: a Children's Oncology Group study. J Clin Oncol 2004;22:2718–2723.
55 Monagle P, Chan A, Massicotte P, Chalmers E, Michelson AD: Antithrombotic therapy in children. Chest 2004;126:645S–687S.
56 Journeycake JM, Buchanan GR: Thrombotic complications of central venous catheters in children. Curr Opin Hematol 2003;10:369–374.

Acta Hæmatologica

Acta Haematol 2006;115:207–213
DOI: 10.1159/000090937

Postthrombotic Syndrome in Children

Marilyn J. Manco-Johnson

Mountain States Regional Hemophilia and Thrombosis Center, Department of Pediatrics, University of Colorado Health Sciences Center and The Children's Hospital, Denver, Colo., USA

Key Words
Postthrombotic syndrome · PTS prevention · PTS therapy · Children · Venous thromboembolism

Abstract
The postthrombotic syndrome (PTS) is a clinical condition of limb pain along with physical findings that range from swelling to stasis ulcers following one or more episodes of deep vein thrombosis (DVT). While venous thromboembolism has recently gained increased recognition in children, the sequelae of limb thrombi are being recognized in a substantial proportion of affected children, and with varying degrees of severity. PTS is caused by both obstructed as well as refluxed venous blood flow, with combined effects of obstruction and reflux resulting in earlier, and more extensive symptoms. PTS can be diagnosed using an evaluation tool adapted from an international adult scale. Certain risk factors predispose children to PTS including elevations in factor VIII activity and D-dimer, clot occlusiveness, clot persistence, number of venous segments involved and duration of observation following DVT. Optimal prevention and treatment have not yet been determined, although antithrombotic therapy to facilitate rapid clot resolution, elevation, compression, moderate exercise and achievement of optimal body weight are likely to improve outcome.

Introduction

Postthrombotic syndrome (PTS) following an episode of venous thromboembolism is a commonly diagnosed condition in middle-aged to older adults. Until recently, PTS was rarely diagnosed in pediatric patients. With increased awareness and improved diagnosis of thrombosis in children, and especially with the development of comprehensive clinical programs to follow cohorts of children following an episode of thrombosis, the clinical spectrum of PTS is becoming delineated. Because children can be expected to live six or more decades following an episode of deep vein thrombosis (DVT), the medical and financial costs of this complication are expected to be disproportionately high in young patients. In addition, aerobic activities including participation in team sports play an important role in normal childhood physical and social development. Thus PTS places a burden on appropriate growth and development in children, as well as imposing limitations of pain and decreased function. As it has such a significant impact on long-term function and cost of care, strategies to prevent or treat PTS in children are extremely important. This paper will review the PTS in pediatric patients including definition, pathophysiology, diagnosis, prevalence, risk factors, therapy and outcome. Finally, unanswered questions and issues for future research will be identified.

KARGER

Fax +41 61 306 12 34
E-Mail karger@karger.ch
www.karger.com

Accessible online at:
www.karger.com/aha

Marilyn J. Manco-Johnson, MD
Mountain States Regional Hemophilia and Thrombosis Center
PO Box 6507, Mail Stop F-416
Aurora, CO 80045-0507 (USA)
Tel. +1 303 724 0365, Fax +1 303 724 0947, E-Mail marilyn.manco-johnson@uchsc.edu

Acute Venous Thrombosis	Effective Preventive Intervention Therapies for Acute Venous Thrombosis
Clot across valve	I. Prompt clot lysis
↓	↓
Venous obstruction, Valve dilatation and damage	Prevention of obstruction and/or Valvular damage
	II. Compressive stockings
↓	↓
Acute → Chronic venous hypertension	Prevention of venous hypertension
	III. Limb elevation
↓	↓
Venous valve incompetence and reflux flow	Prevention of venous valve incompetence and reflux flow
↓	↓
Limb discoloration, swelling and pain (PTS)	Prevention of PTS

Fig. 1. Schemas for the pathophysiology of the PTS and a proposed preventive strategy.

Definition/Pathophysiology

The PTS is a clinical constellation of typical objective and subjective findings following an episode of DVT of the limb [1, 2]. Classically PTS describes the sequelae of DVT in the lower extremity although upper extremities can be similarly involved. PTS manifests primarily with limb swelling and pain that result from both obstructed as well as refluxed blood flow, with additive effects when both reflux resulting from valvular incompetence is present with obstructed flow [1, 3, 4]. The pathophysiology of PTS and a strategy to prevent PTS are shown on figure 1. Partially or completely obstructed flow develops immediately following thrombus formation and may resolve or persist. Clot resolution, particularly early resolution, is related to lower rates of venous hypertension, reflux flow and PTS, while clot persistence is associated with an increased likelihood of PTS [5, 6]. Reflux flow or flow away from the heart resulting in tissue edema of the ankles and calves is caused by damage to the venous valves. Limb swelling from reflux flow is accentuated by prolonged standing and may be accompanied by ruddy discoloration of overlying skin. Reflux flow develops over time following an episode of venous thrombosis, and may increase for at least 1 year [5]. In addition, limb pain and swelling are usual at the time of acute DVT and resolve over days to months. The development of pain and swelling secondary to PTS may overlap that related to the acute DVT. For both of these reasons, PTS cannot reliably be diagnosed until 6 months or more following an episode of DVT, and the possibility of PTS cannot be excluded until 5–10 years following the thrombotic event [2]. Long-term studies needed to determine the prevalence and severity of DVT in infants and children have not yet been conducted in sizable pediatric populations.

Late in the course of PTS, skin overlying edematous tissue becomes indurated and hyperpigmented. The skin discoloration is typically red at the outset and eventually becomes purple or brown. Because of the dryness and scaly characteristics of skin in PTS, this syndrome has been called 'venous eczema'. Eventually the indurated skin breaks down, causing deep open ulcerations of venous stasis that heal poorly.

Fig. 2. A pediatric PTS outcome assessment tool [9]. This tool for PTS, adapted from a validated adult scale, combines physical findings of swelling, visible collaterals, venous eczema and stasis ulcers with an assessment of pain limiting aerobic exercise, activities of daily living and rest.

FUNCTIONAL OUTCOME ASSESSMENT

Race: _______ Gender: ______ Age: _____ Ht: _____ Wt: _____ BMI: _______

Dominant Side: rt ______ lft ______

Circumference in cm

	Right	Left
Thigh		
Calf		
Upper Arm		
Forearm		

CEAP

Physical Findings	**Right Limb Upper/Lower**	**Left Limb Upper/Lower**
1. No visible or palpable signs of venous disease	/	/
2. Swelling, with or without pitting edema	/	/
3. Dilated collateral circulation of extremity only	/	/
4. Skin changes ascribed tovenous disease (i.e., Pigmentation, venous eczema)	/	/
5. Skin changes as in 4 with ulceration	/	/

Use the Wong-Baker Faces Pain Rating Scale below to assess pain for the affected and contralateral limbs. All limbs should be rated 0 to 5 for each level of activity.

Pain Outcome: Wong-Baker (Faces) Scale Right Limb	**Right Limb Upper/Lower**	**Left Limb Upper/Lower**
With aerobic exercise only	/	/
With activities of daily living	/	/
At rest	/	/

If choose yes to pain: does it limit your activities: YES ________ NO ________

Wong-Baker Faces Pain Rating Scale

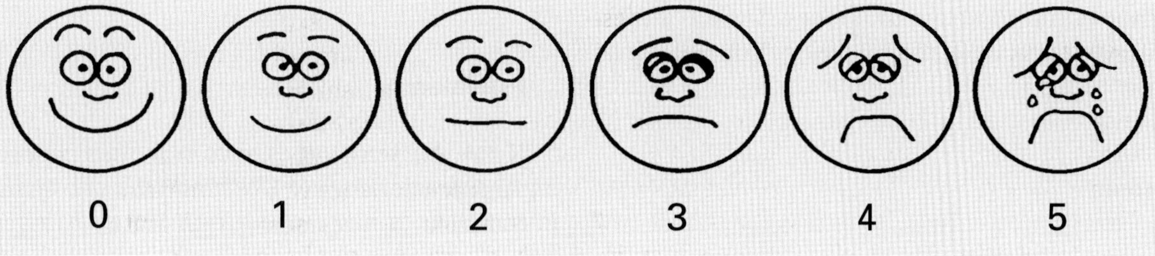

Aerobic exercise only: implies that symptoms are present only when child engages in a vigorous age-appropriate sport such as running, lap swimming, soccer, basketball or volleyball.

Activities of daily living: implies that a child is symptomatic when engaging in ordinary age-appropriate activities in the home, school and community. These symptoms limit and alter a child's ordinary day-to-day activities such as walking at school, shopping with the family or participating in a birthday party.

At rest: implies a constant presence of symptoms that is independent of activity. The child's daily life is severely limited by symptoms.

2

Table 1. Prevalence of PTS in children following an episode of venous thromboembolism

Series	Pediatric patient group	n	Rate of PTS, %
Massicotte et al. [17]	central venous catheters	244	9.5
Monagle et al. [18]	VTE	405	12.4
Häusler et al. [7]	IVC	33	21
Glaser et al. [19]	catheters for cancer	12	25
Journeycake et al. [20]	catheters for hemophilia	8	37.5
Van Ommen et al. [21]	congenital heart disease	28	50
Kuhle et al. [22]	DVT	153	63
Van Ommen et al. [23]	VTE	33	70

VTE = Venous thromboembolism; IVC = inferior vena cava.

Collateral circulation is developed from the formation of new veins shortly after the onset of thrombotic obstruction. Collateral veins lack venous valves and are prone to varicosities and dependent edema. Sometimes abdominal wall collateral veins can be detected in the absence of a history of recognized thrombosis. Prominent collateral vein formation on the trunk may indicate significant silent portal or vena caval obstruction.

Following an episode of thrombosis, fibrin clot may become adherent to the venous wall or the affected vein may become atretic. A series of German children studied years following thrombosis of the inferior vena cava demonstrated the formation of intracaval membranous webs [7]. In an analogous fashion, cavernous transformation of the portal vein, that has been considered a congenital vascular anomaly, may develop from an episode of undetected portal vein thrombosis in infancy. In fact, atresia of the inferior vena cava may develop from previous thrombosis.

Diagnosis

PTS is diagnosed primarily by physical examination. A pediatric PTS scale was adapted from the adult scale of Eklöf et al. [8] and validated in healthy children [9]. A pediatric evaluation instrument for PTS is shown on figure 2; examples of the stages are shown in figure 3a–d. The first stage of PTS is limb swelling, followed by a progression through dilated superficial collateral veins, skin induration and hyperpigmentation and finally, frank ulceration.

Swelling, in addition to pain, is the primary presenting sign of acute DVT. With elevation and compression, swelling will decrease over days to weeks. Swelling also indicates the first stage of venous insufficiency causing PTS with increased venous pressure and dependent collections of pooled interstitial fluid. Extremity swelling should not be attributed to PTS unless it is present 1 year or more following an initial episode of DVT or if swelling develops after initial signs of DVT have completely resolved. Swelling is usually circumferential and can be pitting or nonpitting. Swelling with PTS typically is exaggerated by prolonged standing and improves with limb elevation.

Collateral veins present as development of dilated tortuous superficial vessels. In children collaterals are usually detected on the trunk and the proximal extremity, shoulder or groin. In stage 3 PTS, the color of skin overlying a region of venous insufficiency initially is red, and develops into a brown to purple hyperpigmentation. The skin progressively becomes thickened, dry and scaly, leading to the historic designation, 'venous eczema'. If untreated, skin in stage 3 PTS becomes progressively tight, thinned and shiny. Skin breakdown leads to deep painful venous stasis ulcers, or stage 4 PTS.

While there are no specific tests to diagnose PTS, obstructed and/or reflux flow can be determined as risk factors or supportive evidence of PTS using either plethysmography or ultrasonography [10, 11]. Collateral venous flow can be confirmed using either computerized tomography or magnetic resonance venography with contrast, color Doppler imaging or radionuclide venography [12–16]. Doppler techniques are more commonly helpful in the neck and superior vena cava, whereas CT or MRI are often more helpful in the pelvis.

Prevalence

Relatively few studies have evaluated children following an episode of acute DVT, and the prevalence of PTS in these series has ranged from 9.5 to 70% [7, 17–22]. Table 1 displays published results. Although the reasons for the wide range of prevalence are not completely clear, the rate of PTS appears to increase with time in children, similar to results reported in adults. Controlled prospective studies are needed to determine the true incidence of PTS in children following an episode of venous thromboembolism.

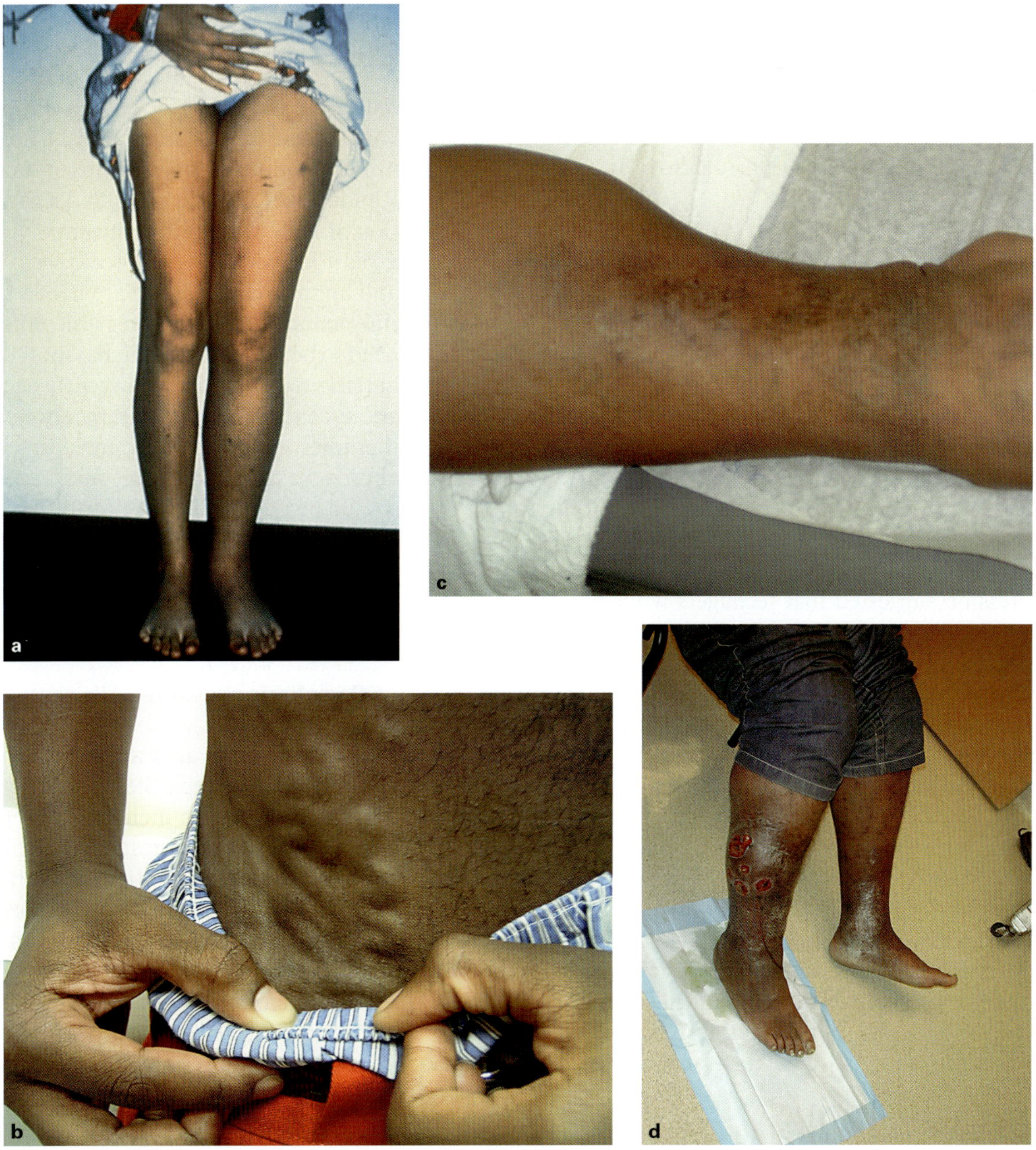

Fig. 3. PTS grading system [8]: grade 1, extremity swelling (**a**), grade 2, dilated superficial collateral vessels (**b**), grade 3, venous eczema with skin dryness, induration and hyperpigmentation (**c**), and grade 4, venous stasis ulcers (**d**).

Risk Factors

Investigations of the risk factors for PTS development in children are in their infancy. Risk factors determined to date for pediatric PTS are shown on table 2, and include elevations of factor VIII and/or D-dimer at the time of presentation and at 3–6 months following an episode of thrombosis, clot that occludes a vessel, lack of clot resolution, number of vessels involved with thrombosis, and duration of follow-up [9, 21, 23]. However, in one series, most children with signs and symptoms of PTS were found to have complete resolution of the venous thrombosis and no symptomatic child had reflux of venous blood flow [21].

Table 2. Risk factors for PTS in pediatric patients

Elevations in factor VIII and/or D-dimer at the time of presentation with VTE
Elevations in factor VIII and/or D-dimer 3–6 months following VTE
Clot that completely occludes the affected vein
Clot persistence
Number of vessels involved
Duration of follow-up
Increased body mass index?

Increased body mass index has been associated with an increased risk of PTS in adults [24]. While we have observed an increased body mass index in all of our adolescent patients with grades 3 and 4 PTS (unpubl. data), formal studies relating body mass index with PTS in pediatric patients are still lacking. While our clinical impression suggested that teenagers with the lupus anticoagulant were at high risk for PTS, statistical analysis did not support either adolescent age or the lupus anticoagulant as independent risk factors [9]. Other factors predictive of PTS risk in adults include recurrent thrombosis, increased age, female gender, hormonal therapy, varicose veins and abdominal surgery [25, 26].

Decreased PTS risk is predicted by early clot resolution with thrombolysis or mechanical clot disruption, use of compressive stockings and secondary prophylaxis against thrombus recurrence [26]. Individually tailored graduated compressive stockings, e.g. Jobst stockings, with 30–35 mm Hg compression appear to be more effective than simpler alternatives. Adolescents in particular are loath to display a visible sign of disability, and this aversion is a barrier to compliance with use of compression stockings.

Therapy for Established PTS

Standard therapies for stage 1 and 2 PTS include use of compression stockings, limb elevation, avoidance of prolonged standing, and alternating limb weight bearing. Recently, weight loss and mild exercise have been explored as treatments for PTS [27, 28]. Therapy for advanced PTS is very difficult; venous stasis ulcerations tend to be chronic and recurrent. Intermittent compression boots, venous stripping, topical hydrophilic therapies and other local therapies are usually employed. Stasis ulcers can be managed by dermatologists, surgeons or burn teams and local expertise dictates referral patterns.

Future Directions

Most aspects of PTS in children require additional data. The incidence of PTS in children, relationship to various risk factors and natural history need to be determined on multiple populations of representative patients. Randomized clinical trials to determine optimal prevention of PTS using initial thrombolysis, long-term anticoagulation, compression stockings, weight management and appropriate exercise are needed. The efficacy of initial therapies including rest, elevation and compression need to be documented. Behavioral research to overcome barriers to compliance is urgently needed, particularly for adolescents. There is a tremendous need for improved therapies for severe PTS, including stasis ulcers. Newer approaches to surgical reconstruction of venous valves should be pursued [29]. Future efforts to treat venous stasis ulcers may focus on the delivery of oxygen and nutrients to ischemic tissue by promoting neovascularization via angiogenic factors.

Conclusion

Children of all ages are at risk for PTS following an episode of DVT, regardless of the site or trigger of initial thrombus. Although incidence and risk factors have not been definitively determined, there is mounting data that children suffer substantial morbidity following venous thrombosis that interferes with normal-age appropriate activity and quality of life, as well as predisposing to progressive venous disease. Research efforts should be directed to understand the pathophysiology and treatment of PTS in children in order to limit severity of disease and improve long-term outcome.

Acknowledgements

This project was funded by grants No. U27/CCU812106 from the Centers for Disease Control and Prevention and 5 M01 RR00069, General Clinical Research Centers Program, National Center for Research Resources, NIH.

References

1 Comerota AJ: Thrombolytic therapy for acute deep vein thrombosis; in Comerota AJ (eds): Thrombolytic Therapy for Acute Vascular Disease. Philadelphia, Lippincott, 1995, pp 175–195.

2 Prandoni P, Lensing A, Cogo A, Cuppini S, Villalta S, Carta M, Cattelan AM, Polistena P, Bernardi E, Prins MH: The long-term clinical course of acute deep venous thrombosis. Ann Intern Med 1996;125:1–7.

3 Shull KC, Nicolaides AN, Fernandes e Fernandeo J, Miles C, Horner J, Needham T, Cooke ED, Eastcott FH: Significance of popliteal reflux in relation to ambulatory venous pressure and ulceration. Arch Surg 1979;114:1304–1306.

4 Franzeck UK, Schalch I, Bollinger A: On the relationship between changes in the deep veins evaluated by duplex sonography and the postthrombotic syndrome 12 years after deep vein thrombosis. Thromb Haemost 1997;77:1109–1112.

5 Markel A, Manzo R, Bergelin R, Standness E: Valvular reflux after deep vein thrombosis: incidence and time of occurrence. J Vasc Surg 1979;15:377–384.

6 Meissner MH, Manzo RA, Gergelin RO, Markel A, Strandness DE: Deep venous insufficiency: the relationship between lysis and subsequent reflux. J Vasc Surg 1993;18:596–608.

7 Häusler M, Hübner D, Delhaas T, Mühler EG: Long term complications of inferior vena cava thrombosis. Arch Dis Child 2001;85:228–233.

8 Eklöf B, Rutherford RB, Bergan JJ, Carpentier PH, Gloviczki P, Kistner RL, et al: Revision of the CEAP classification for chronic venous disorders: consensus statement. J Vasc Surg 2004;40:1248–1252.

9 Manco-Johnson MJ, Knapp-Clevenger R, Miller B, Hays T: Post-thrombotic syndrome (PTS) in children: validation of a new pediatric outcome instrument and results in a comprehensive cohort of children with extremity deep vein thrombosis (DVT). Blood 2003;102:553a.

10 O'Donnell TF Jr, McEnroe CS, Heggerick P: Chronic venous insufficiency. Surg Clin North Am 1990;70:159–180.

11 Welch HJ, Faliakou EC, McLaughlin RL, Umphrey SE, Belkin M, O'Donnell TF Jr: Comparison of descending phlebography with quantitative photoplethysmography, air plethysmography, and duplex quantitative valve closure time in assessing deep venous reflux. J Vasc Surg 1992;16:913–920.

12 Umeoka S, Koyama T, Togashi K, Kobayashi H, Akuta K: Vascular dilatation in the pelvis: identification with CT and MR imaging. Radiographics 2004;24:193–208.

13 Yoshizako T, Sugimura K, Kawamitsu H, Yoshikawa K: Two-dimensional time-of-flight MR venography: assessment with detection of chronic deep venous thrombosis in combination with magnetization transfer contrast. J Comput Assist Tomography 1996;20:957–964.

14 Tighe DA, Paul JJ, Huhta JC: Superior vena caval syndrome: color flow Doppler detection of collateral venous channels. J Am Soc Echocardiogr 2000;13:780–784.

15 Conkbayir I, Men S, Yanik B, Hekimoglu B: Color Doppler sonographic finding of retrograde jugular venous flow as a sign of innominate vein occlusion. J Clin Ultrasound 2002;30:392–398.

16 Mahmud AM, Isawa T, Teshima T, Hirano T, Anazawa Y, Miki M, Nukiwa T: Radionuclide venography and its functional analysis in superior vena cava syndrome. J Nucl Med 1996;37:1460–1464.

17 Massicotte MP, Dix D, Monagle P, Adams M, Andrew M: Central venous catheter related thrombosis in children: analysis of the Canadian Registry of Venous Thromboembolic Complications. J Pediatr 1998;133:770–776.

18 Monagle P, Adams M, Mahoney M, Ali K, Barnard D, Bernstein M, Brisson L, David M, Desai S, Scully MF, Halton J, Israels S, Jardine L, Leaker M, McCusker P, Silva M, Wu J, Anderson R, Andrew M, Massicotte MP: Outcome of pediatric thromboembolic disease: a report of the Canadian Childhood Thrombophilia Registry. Pediatr Res 2000;47:763–766.

19 Glaser DW, Medeiros D, Rollins N, Buchanan GR: Catheter-related thrombosis in children with cancer. J Pediatr 2001;138:255–259.

20 Journeycake JM, Quinn CT, Miller KL, Zajac JL, Buchanan GR: Catheter-related deep venous thrombosis in children with hemophilia. Blood 2001;98:1727–1731.

21 van Ommen CH, Ottenkamp J, Lam J, Brennickmeier M, Heijmans HAS, Büller HR, Peters M: The risk of postthrombotic syndrome in children with congenital heart disease. J Pediatr 2002;141:582–586.

22 Kuhle S, Koloshuk B, MarzinottoV, Bauman M, Massicotte P, Andrew M, Chan A, Abdolell M, Mitchell L: A cross-sectional study evaluating post-thrombotic syndrome in children. Thromb Res 2003;111:227–233.

23 van Ommen CH, Heijboer H, van den Dool EJ, Hutten BA, Peters M: Pediatric venous thromboembolic disease in one single center: congenital prothrombotic disorders and the clinical outcome. J Thromb Haemost 2003;1:2516–2522.

24 Goldenberg NA, Knapp-Clevenger R, Manco-Johnson MJ: Elevated plasma factor VIII and D-dimer levels as predictors of poor outcomes of thrombosis in children. N Engl J Med 2004;351:1081–1088.

25 Ageno W, Piantanida E, Dentali F, Steidl L, Mera V, Squizzato A, Marchesi C, Venco A: Body mass index is associated with the development of the post-thrombotic syndrome. Thromb Haemost 2003;89:305–309.

26 Kahn SR, Ginsberg JS: Relationship between deep venous thrombosis and the postthrombotic syndrome. Arch Intern Med 2004;164:17–26.

27 Raymond LW: Getting a leg up on the postthrombotic syndrome. Chest 2003;123:327–330.

28 Kahn SR, Azoulay L, Hirsch A, Haber M, Strulovitch C, Shrier I: Acute effects of exercise in patients with previous deep venous thrombosis. Impact of the postthrombotic syndrome. Chest 2003;123:399–405.

29 Maleti O: Venous valvular reconstruction in post-thrombotic syndrome. A new technique. J Mal Vasc 2002;27:218–221.

Acta Haematologica

Acta Haematol 2006;115:214–220
DOI: 10.1159/000090938

Exercise-Induced Deep Vein Thrombosis of the Upper Extremity

1. Literature Review

Leonardo R. Brandão[a] Suzan Williams[a] Walter H.A. Kahr[a] Clodagh Ryan[a] Michael Temple[b] Anthony K.C. Chan[c,d]

[a]Division of Haematology/Oncology, Department of Paediatrics, [b]Department of Diagnostic Imaging, Centre for Image Guided Therapy and [c]Department of Paediatric Laboratory Medicine, The Hospital for Sick Children, Toronto; [d]Department of Paediatrics, McMaster University, Hamilton, Canada

Key Words

Venous thrombosis · Upper extremity · Effort-related · Post-thrombotic syndrome · Children

Abstract

Paget-Schroetter syndrome or effort-related upper extremity deep vein thrombosis is a rare condition that usually afflicts young healthy individuals, most commonly males. The cause is multifactorial but almost always involves extrinsic compression of the subclavian vein at the thoracic inlet, causing venous stenosis from repetitive trauma. The diagnosis of this condition may be difficult, and its delay may contribute to potential complications including thrombosis progression, pulmonary embolism, thrombosis recurrence, and post-thrombotic syndrome. Similarly, the best therapeutic option has not been established and in the lack of evidence-based guidelines, treatment may be extremely challenging especially in children, in whom long-term complications can be particularly disabling.

Introduction

Venous thromboembolic events (VTEs) are recognized as a growing clinical problem in children. The incidence and epidemiology of VTEs has been described in prospective population-based studies reported by international registries (i.e. Canadian, German and Dutch) [1–4], which revealed the presence of at least one associated underlying medical condition in most cases. Among all registries, the presence of a central venous line (CVL) was the most common etiologic factor. For this reason, in contrast to adults, the upper venous system is involved in more than 50% of VTEs in children due to the presence of CVLs [1, 4]. Spontaneous VTEs are rare in children, and they usually involve the renal veins in the neonatal period or the lower extremity venous system in the nonneonatal age group [1–4]. However, effort-related upper-extremity deep vein thrombosis (UEDVT) or Paget-Schroetter syndrome is a form of spontaneous upper-extremity VTE, which has not been well characterized in children.

Over a century after the original description of Paget-Schroetter syndrome, controversy regarding its diagnosis, management, and outcome persists. The resultant lack of large reported series and of comparative clinical trials is most likely responsible for the widespread uncertainty

KARGER

Fax +41 61 306 12 34
E-Mail karger@karger.ch
www.karger.com

0001–5792/06/1154–0214$23.50/0

Accessible online at:
www.karger.com/aha

Leonardo R. Brandão, MD
The Hospital for Sick Children, 555 University Avenue, Black Wing, Room 10412
Toronto, Ont. M5G 1X8 (Canada)
Tel. +1 416 813 7500, ext. 5401, Fax +1 416 813 5327
E-Mail leonardo.brandao@sickkids.ca

over many aspects of this condition. This article will be published in two complementary parts. The first part will review the available information of this condition most commonly found in adults, focusing on its epidemiology, clinical presentation, diagnostic methods, therapeutic options, and outcome, setting up the stage for a more critical reading of the second part. The second half will report the first series containing only patients within the pediatric range who were diagnosed with effort-related UEDVT [5].

History

Activity-induced or effort-related thrombosis of the subclavian and/or axillary veins is a special form of venous thrombosis distinct from classical deep vein thrombosis (DVT) of the lower extremity and probably from CVL-induced UEDVT. It was first described by Jean Cruveilhier (1791–1873), but not as the entity is recognized today. His description was followed by two others. (1) In 1875 in London, Sir James Paget [6] hypothesized about the presence of spontaneous thrombosis of the veins draining the upper extremity, which he described in patients with acute pain and swelling of the arm and named 'gouty phlebitis'. (2) In 1884 in Vienna, von Schroetter [7] reported a similar case occurring in an otherwise healthy painter who was working at the time of onset. It was the physician's feeling that the axillary vein was directly damaged by repetitive stretching that resulted from muscular strain. In 1934, Matas [8] introduced this condition to the North American medical literature and in 1948, Hughes [9] coined the term Paget-Schroetter syndrome when he described this condition in a review of 320 cases [10]. In 1966, the terminology 'effort-related' thrombosis emerged [11] in recognition of the impression that strenuous use of the arm and/or shoulder in physically active patients was correlated with UEDVT. Since 1966, there have been 744 patients reported in 7 literature reviews, 15 case series, and 24 case reports. This syndrome may be even rarer in children, and its incidence, epidemiology, and clinical outcome have not been reported in a series containing only pediatric patients.

Upper Venous System Anatomy

Veins in the arm drain via the basilic or cephalic system. The basilic vein flows into the axillary vein, which is joined by the cephalic vein to form the subclavian vein

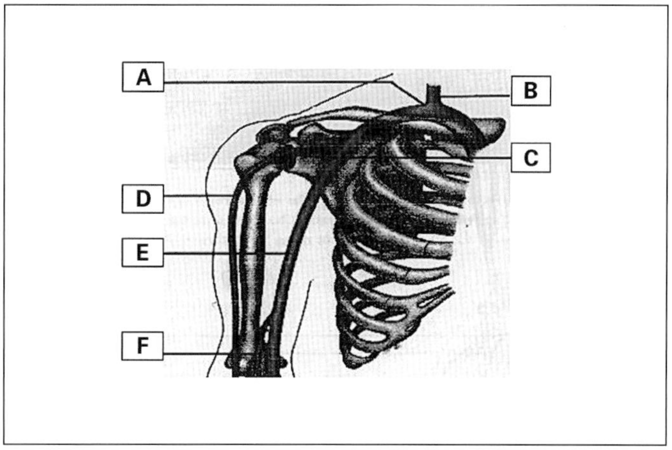

Fig. 1. Anatomy of the veins of the upper limb: venous angle (junction of subclavian vein and internal jugular vein; A), internal jugular vein (B), axillary vein (C), cephalic vein (D), brachial vein (E), and basilic vein (F) [12].

(fig. 1) [12]. The axillary vein is contiguous to the basilic vein, traveling the tunnel formed by the clavicle and subclavian muscle anteriorly, the scalene muscle laterally, the first rib posterior-inferiorly, and the costoclavicular ligament medially. From the subscapular region, the axillary vein receives subscapular and suprascapular veins (not depicted in fig. 1). There are many anastomotic collateral pathways that can potentially bypass the axillary-subclavian venous region. They are divided as follows: (1) shoulder to chest wall, (2) shoulder to ipsilateral anterior neck, (3) shoulder to ipsilateral posterior neck, and (4) shoulder to contralateral neck. In the event of axillary vein thrombosis, collaterals will usually develop from the shoulder to the chest wall, whereas in thrombosis of the subclavian vein, collaterals will generally develop to the ipsilateral posterior neck or from the shoulder to the contralateral neck [13]. Recognition of the collateral pathways allows proper interpretation of clinical and imaging findings in UEDVT.

Pathophysiology

Thoracic outlet syndrome (TOS) refers to compression of the neurovascular bundle, including the brachial plexus, subclavian artery, and subclavian vein as it exits the thoracic inlet, delimited by the scalene muscles, the clavicle, and the first rib. Cervical ribs, musculofascial bands, and clavicular or first rib abnormalities have also been described as other causes for TOS [14]. Symptoms include a combination of vascular and neurologic findings. In pediatrics, TOS is very rare, and its management is controversial, varying from a conservative nonoperative management with shoulder-strengthening exercises to surgery [15, 16].

In Paget-Schroetter syndrome, the vein is repeatedly compressed either as it exits in the thoracic inlet or in the costoclavicular space. Abduction of the upper limbs, cervical extension, and dropping of the shoulders promotes narrowing of this space. Repetitive microtrauma to the vessel wall results in fibrous tissue formation that permanently strangles the vein, predisposing it to thrombosis. The temporary elevation of the levels of some coagulation components (i.e. factor VIII and von Willebrand factor) during exercise represents another theoretical risk factor. During strenuous exercise, this rise may contribute to a transient hypercoagulable state, leading to thrombus formation within the area of abnormal blood flow.

Venous thrombi are formed in the milieu of low flow and low shear stress, consisting mainly of fibrin strands, red blood cells, and few platelets. In general, the thrombus will originate in the valve pockets, growing to its ultimate site depending on the three elements defined in the Virchow's triad (blood flow, vessel wall, and blood coagulability).

Postthrombotic syndrome (PTS) develops as a result of venous hypertension due to persistent outflow obstruction secondary to thrombus formation or to venous valve incompetence, or both. Long-standing venous hypertension leads to the onset of valve incompetence at the level of collateral perforating veins. The destruction of the valve system allows transmission of the high pressure from the deep venous system to the superficial venous system and subsequently to the subcutaneous capillaries, resulting in increased endothelial permeability. Leakage of large molecules at the capillary bed will result in local edema, hyperpigmentation, and ulcer formation. During an acute thrombotic event, presentation with early edema is suggestive of blood flow obstruction; late onset limb edema is suggestive of valve incompetence. Increased venous pressure is generated by long standing or walking on the lower limbs in cases of leg DVT, or by effort-related activity of the upper limb in Paget-Schroetter syndrome, which will continue to promote the injury mechanism towards PTS development. As a result of the increased reversed pressure gradient in the venous bed, there is reduction of the capillary flow with local trapping of white blood cells and release of proteolytic enzymes, with subsequent ulcer formation.

The role of thrombophilia in effort-related UEDVT is unknown. Heron et al. [17] reported 51 adult patients, comparing the incidence of thrombophilia between effort-related episodes (20 patients) with primary UEDVT. Among the 20 patients with effort-related VTE, only 1 had factor V (FV) Leiden without positive family history, and 2 patients had positive anticardiolipin on one occasion (intermittent lupus antibodies were found in our series). Their conclusion was that hypercoagulable states appear to play a role in idiopathic, but not in effort-related UEDVT.

A second similar study from Argentina compared 31 adult patients distributed between effort-related UEDVT and primary UEDVT. The authors found a high incidence of thrombophilia in both groups, but no difference between the groups [18]. Nineteen patients (61.3%) had at least one thrombophilia abnormality, distributed as follows: (1) 31% lupus anticoagulant (LA), (2) 20% prothrombin G20210A gene mutation (PT G20210A), (3) 16.1% high homocysteine (HCY) level, (4) 12.9% anticardiolipin, (5) 12.9% factor V (FV) Leiden, and (6) 4.7% protein S defect.

Martinelli et al. [19] reported on 115 primary UEDVTs (including 25% effort-related VTEs) and 797 healthy controls with a follow-up of 5.1 years. The adjusted odds ratio for UEDVT was 6.2 (95% CI 2.5–15.7) for FV Leiden, 5.0 (95% CI 2.0–12.2) for PT G20210A, and 4.9 (95% CI 1.1–22.0) for the anticoagulant protein deficiencies. The recurrence rate was 4.4% patient-years in patients with thrombophilia and 1.6% patient-years in those without it. No comparison between effort-related and primary UEDVT was done in this last study. Overall, the contribution of thrombophilic states to effort-related UEDVT in adult patients is less in comparison to idiopathic UEDVT.

Incidence and Definitions

Primary or spontaneous UEDVT is a rare disorder, with an incidence reported in adults of 2 per 100,000 persons per year [20], accounting for 11 in 100,000 US hospital admissions [21]. In adults, primary subclavian-axillary vein thrombosis corresponds to approximately 2–4% of all thrombotic episodes [20–24], comprising approximately 30% of all cases of UEDVT [25]. Primary UEDVT is classified as either idiopathic UEDVT, or as effort-related UEDVT, the latter being also called Paget-Schroetter syndrome. Historically, this was considered a benign and self-limited condition [26, 27]; however, more recent reports have not confirmed this initial impression.

Clinical Presentation

Paget-Schroetter syndrome or effort-related UEDVT is often referred to as spontaneous due to its unexpected presentation in healthy, generally young (early 30s) individuals [28]. The literature reports a 2:1 predilection of males over females, with 75% of patients reporting an antecedent event of strenuous or repetitive activity before the presentation. The dominant extremity is involved in 60–80% of cases. Within the neurovascular bundle, nerves and veins are at anatomical opposite ends of the thoracic outlet. Therefore, compression of the neurovascular bundle leading to subclavian-axillary vein thrombosis has associated neurologic symptoms in only 4–10% of patients. Symptoms of arterial and/or neurologic compression are more common manifestations of TOS.

The typical feature of primary UEDVT is swelling of the involved extremity. The edema characteristically involves the entire arm and hand and is usually nonpitting. Pain can be present, being described as a 'feeling of tightness' that usually worsens with exertion. Mild cyanosis with or without a palpable cord can also be found at presentation. The majority of patients probably develop venous stenosis slowly, seeking medical attention only when the thrombus size increases to a dimension that impedes venous return, causing symptoms. An indeterminate number of patients never seek medical attention because of the development of adequate collateral circulation. However, even after treatment, some of the collateral vessels will still be submitted to impingement through the thoracic inlet, resulting in different degrees of residual symptoms.

Diagnosis

Suspicion of UEDVT is raised in cases of relatively sudden onset arm swelling, pain, and/or venous engorgement. Symptoms are usually present within the first 24 h of the triggering event, but partial venous occlusions can cause a delay in presentation and diagnosis. Objective documentation of the presence of thrombus can be obtained by duplex ultrasonography examination, venography, and by other noninvasive imaging modalities, such as magnetic resonance angiography or computerized tomography (CT). In a prospective case-control study done by Prandoni et al. [29] to assess the diagnostic accuracy of imaging, only 27 of 58 patients with initial clinical findings suggestive of UEDVT who underwent venography had their thrombotic events confirmed. This result underlines the necessity to confirm or exclude clinically suspected UEDVT with objective tests.

Venography is still the 'gold standard' in evaluating subclavian-axillary vein thrombosis, but its interpretation can be challenging. Positioning of the patients' upper extremities is crucial; they should be abducted at least 30° to demonstrate compression. Positive findings reveal various degrees of venous occlusion or stenosis and the extent of local collateral circulation. A limitation to this test is that a significant percentage of the normal population may present with an abnormal finding during extreme arm abduction [30].

CT and magnetic resonance imaging (MRI) are not routinely obtained because they have not yet been shown to have an impact on therapeutic decisions or outcome. However, helical CT and MRI venography and/or magnetic resonance angiography can also be used to diagnose UEDVT. While both methods seem to correlate well with the anatomic and functional assessment of the thoracic outlet region [31–33], MRI may fail to detect the presence of subclavian thrombi [34].

Treatment and Complications

Therapy of primary UEDVT was initially based on rest and elevation of the affected limb with or without systemic anticoagulation. The concept of venous patency restoration and/or extrinsic decompression became increasingly accepted as a new therapeutic approach after it became clear that the underlying etiology of this entity is venous compression. In the last decade, conscrvative anticoagulation therapy has been losing ground to more aggressive treatment modalities. Thrombectomy, thrombolytic therapy (systemic or catheter-directed), balloon angioplasty followed by stenting, and thoracic outlet decompression were applied and reported in different small case series, but the best therapeutic approach has not yet been established.

After recovery from the acute event, most active patients may still have residual symptoms. These findings, unlike lower extremity DVT symptoms, may correlate to residual obstruction rather than reflux. Patients complain of pain and swelling that are made worse by arm activity. Recurrent disabling symptoms may occur in up to 75% of patients. However, stasis dermatitis and ulceration are almost never seen in UEDVT [35]. Venous gangrene is another extremely rare complication of UEDVT. It is estimated that upper-extremity phlegmasia cerulea dolens constitutes 2–5% of all phlegmasia cases [36]. The cases reported were all secondary to an underlying hypercoagulable state or cancer. To date, there have been no reports of phlegmasia arising from effort-related UEDVT.

Regarding pulmonary embolism (PE), most studies that reported their incidence have grouped primary and secondary UEDVT together. It is difficult to calculate if each UEDVT modality has a different PE incidence rate, but Hughes [10] reported only three cases of PE from his 320 patients. On the other hand, Harley et al. [37] reported an incidence of PE in 10–12% of their patients.

In another recent review on management of UEDVT, Hicken and Ameli [38] compared the number of patients with persistent symptoms grouped by type of treatment. From a total of 304 patients, the incidence of persistent symptoms found in patients treated conservatively (n = 50), with anticoagulation (n = 133), with thrombolysis (n = 31), with surgery and thrombolysis (n = 67), surgery alone (n = 19), or others were respectively: 52, 32, 26, 19, 16 and 50%. These findings suggest that a more aggressive therapy confers a better prognosis in terms of long-term morbidity. However, these numbers originated from separate studies and patient selection bias is possible.

There is consensus among vascular surgeons that early diagnosis followed by intervention provides the most favorable results [39, 40]. Opinions differ, however, in terms of the best fibrinolytic agent used (i.e. urokinase vs. tissue plasminogen activator vs. streptokinase), and the most appropriate timing for the use of fibrinolytic therapy. There is even more controversy regarding the necessity of subsequent surgery after thrombolysis.

In 1993, Machleder [41] proposed delaying the first rib resection until 3 months after thrombolysis. Two years later, Molina [42] was one of the defenders of early surgical intervention immediately after fibrinolysis. More recently, two groups compared both approaches concluding that early surgical intervention provided superior clinical results [43, 44]. In a more conservative approach, only patients remaining with symptoms after 1 month of oral anticoagulation would be considered for surgery [45]. The patients from this series would continue to receive anticoagulation for 4 weeks after the surgical procedure, which would be discontinued after objective confirmation of venous patency [45].

When surgery is indicated, most authors agree that scalenectomy, first rib resection, and thrombolysis should be performed at the same time. The surgical access can be done by either a supraclavicular or a transaxillary approach.

The largest retrospective series in UEDVT therapy over a 30-year experience was published by Urschel and Razzuk [46], including 294 patients with 312 UEDVTs, 18 being bilateral. From this series, the management of UEDVTs was grouped as follows: (1) group I included 35 extremities (11%) treated initially with anticoagulants followed by first rib resection in 20 symptomatic cases, (2) group II included 36 extremities (11.5%) treated with thrombolytic therapy initially, followed by surgery in 20 cases after returning to work, (3) group III included 199 extremities (64%) seen within 4–6 weeks of diagnosis and treated with fibrinolysis plus prompt surgery, and (4) group IV included 42 extremities (13.5%) also treated with clot lysis and prompt surgery done 6 weeks from the time of venous occlusion. From the comparison of all groups, the best results regarding venous patency and clinical improvement was found in group III. Despite receiving the same treatment as group III, none of the 42 extremities treated 6 weeks after the initial VTE could be completely recanalized. Notably, in group IV, of the 35 (100%) extremities that were initially treated solely with anticoagulants (heparin followed by warfarin), 26 (74%) had a recurrent UEDVT and 21 (60%) had long-term morbidity despite surgery. Unfortunately, the authors did not specify the intensity nor the duration of the anticoagulation used in group I. The article also lacks information on how PTS was assessed and the mean patient follow-up of each group. Group I included patients diagnosed before 1980, whereas the other groups were treated after 1980.

Thrombosis of the upper extremity has distinct characteristics in comparison to VTE of the lower limb. A recent survey by the American DVT Registry Database, which enrolled 5,451 consecutive adult patients with acute DVT from October 2001 to March 2002, reported 592 (approximately 11%) patients with UEDVT [47]. The database included both CVL-related UEDVT (6% of total number of cases), non-CVL-related UEDVT (5% of total number of cases), and lower limb DVT (LLDVT; 89% of total number of cases). Effort-related UEDVT was included with the non-CVL-related UEDVT, but the number of cases and their percentage were not specified. In comparison with patients with LLDVT, UEDVT patients were younger (59.2 ± 18.2 vs. 64.2 ± 16.9 years; $p < 0.0001$), less often white (65 vs. 73%; $p < 0.01$), leaner (BMI 26.8 ± 7.1 vs. 28.5 ± 7.3 kg/m^2; $p < 0.0001$), more frequently presented with edema (79 vs. 69%; $p = 0.001$), and less commonly with extremity discomfort (46 vs. 55%; $p < 0.01$), dyspnea, or chest pain. Patients with UEDVT also had symptomatic PE less frequently (3 vs. 16%; $p < 0.001$). For all categories, most patients were treated with 'classic' anticoagulant therapy consisting of

LMWH with transition to warfarin. Catheter-directed or systemic fibrinolysis was rarely used, implemented in only 4% of the non-CVL-related UEDVT and 1% of LLDVT (p = 0.002). Data on clinical outcome was not available from this report.

Conclusion

UEDVT is a serious thrombotic event with potential acute and long-term complications. It is associated with PE and with a high incidence of PTS [27].

Despite the advances in terms of diagnosis, management of exercise-induced UEDVT remains highly controversial. Recently, literature from cardiovascular surgeons suggests that earlier diagnosis and appropriate aggressive intervention leads to better results. However, a proper comparison with 'classic anticoagulation' therapy has not been conducted. Because of the epidemiological characteristics of this entity, an exclusive pediatric series has not been reported in the literature to date.

Acknowledgments

We wish to thank Dr. Fred Pluthero and Ms. Lu Ann Brooker for their critical review of the manuscript. Anthony K.C. Chan is a recipient of a Career Investigator Award from the Heart and Stroke Foundation of Canada.

References

1 Andrew M, David M, Adams M, Ali K, Anderson R, Barnard D, Bernstein M, Brisson L, Cairney B, DeSai D: Venous thromboembolic complications (VTE) in children: first analyses of the Canadian Registry of VTE. Blood 1994; 83:1251–1257.
2 Nowak-Gottl U, von Kries R, Gobel U: Neonatal symptomatic thromboembolism in Germany: two year survey. Arch Dis Child Fetal Neonatal Ed 1997;76:F163–F167.
3 van Ommen CH, Heijboer H, Buller HR, Hirasing RA, Heijmans HS, Peters M: Venous thromboembolism in childhood: a prospective two-year registry in The Netherlands. J Pediatr 2001;139:676–681.
4 Schmidt B, Andrew M: Neonatal thrombosis: report of a prospective Canadian and international registry. Pediatrics 1995;96:939–943.
5 Brandão LR, Williams S, Kahr WHA, Ryan C, Temple M, Chan AKC: Exercise-induced deep vein thrombosis of the upper extremity. 2. A case series in children. Acta Haematol 2006; 115:221–229.
6 Paget J: Clinical Lectures and Essays. London, Longmans Green, 1875.
7 von Schroetter L: Erkrankungen der Gefässe. Nothnagel Handbuch der Pathologie und Therapie. Vienna, Holder, 1884.
8 Matas R: Primary thrombosis of the axillary vein caused by strain. Am J Surg 1934;24:642–656.
9 Hughes ES: Venous obstruction in the upper extremity. Br J Surg 1948;36:155.
10 Hughes ES: Venous obstruction in upper extremity (Paget-Schroetter's syndrome). Review of 320 cases. Int Abstr Surg 1949;88:89–127.
11 Drapanas T, Curran WL: Thrombectomy in the treatment of 'effort' thrombosis of the axillary and subclavian veins. J Trauma 1966;6: 107–119.
12 Rohen JW, Yokochi C, Romrell LJ: Colour Atlas of Anatomy: a Photographic Study of the Human Body, ed 3. New York, Igaku-Shoin, 1993.
13 Richard HM 3rd, Selby JB Jr, Gay SB, Tegtmeyer CJ: Normal venous anatomy and collateral pathways in upper extremity venous thrombosis. Radiographics 1992;12:527–534.
14 Makhoul RG, Machleder HI: Developmental anomalies at the thoracic outlet: an analysis of 200 consecutive cases. J Vasc Surg 1992;16: 534–542.
15 Vercellio G, Baraldini V, Gatti C, Coletti M, Cipolat L: Thoracic outlet syndrome in paediatrics: clinical presentation, surgical treatment, and outcome in a series of eight children. J Pediatr Surg 2003;38:58–61.
16 Yang J, Letts M: Thoracic outlet syndrome in children. J Pediatr Orthop 1996;16:514–517.
17 Heron E, Lozinguez O, Alhenc-Gelas M, Emmerich J, Fiessinger JN: Hypercoagulable states in primary upper-extremity deep vein thrombosis. Arch Intern Med 2000;160:382–386.
18 Hendler MF, Meschengieser SS, Blanco AN, Alberto MF, Salviu MJ, Gennari L, Lazzari MA: Primary upper-extremity deep vein thrombosis: high prevalence of thrombophilic defects. Am J Hematol 2004;76:330–337.
19 Martinelli I, Battaglioli T, Bucciarelli P, Passamonti SM, Mannucci PM: Risk factors and recurrence rate of primary deep vein thrombosis of the upper extremities. Circulation 2004; 110:566–570.
20 Lindblad B, Tengborn L, Bergqvist D: Deep vein thrombosis of the axillary-subclavian veins: epidemiologic data, effects of different types of treatment and late sequelae. Eur J Vasc Surg 1988;2:161–165.
21 Coon WW, Willis PW 3rd: Thrombosis of axillary and subclavian veins. Arch Surg 1967;94: 657–663.
22 Barker NW, Nygaard KK, Walters W: Statistical study of postoperative venous thrombosis and pulmonary embolism. Location of thrombosis; relation of thrombosis and embolism. Proc Staff Meet Mayo Clin 1941;16:33.
23 Ochsner A, DeBakey M, DeCamp PT: Thromboembolism: analysis of cases at Charity Hospital in New Orleans over a 12-year period. Arch Surg 1951;134:405.
24 Martin M: PHLEKO-/PHLEFI-Studien. Vasa 1997;S49:1–39.
25 Mustafa S, Stein PD, Patel KC, Otten TR, Holmes R, Silbergleit A: Upper extremity deep venous thrombosis. Chest 2003;123:1953–1956.
26 Ameli FM, Minas T, Weiss M, Provan JL: Consequences of 'conservative' conventional management of axillary vein thrombosis. Can J Surg 1987;30:167–169.
27 Tilney ML, Griffiths HJ, Edwards EA: Natural history of major venous thrombosis of the upper extremity. Arch Surg 1970;101:792–796.
28 Hurlbert SN, Rutherford RB: Primary subclavian-axillary vein thrombosis. Ann Vasc Surg 1995;9:217–223.
29 Prandoni P, Polistena P, Bernardi E, Cogo A, Casara D, Verlato F, Angelini F, Simioni P, Signorini GP, Benedetti L, Girolami A: Upper-extremity deep vein thrombosis. Risk factors, diagnosis, and complications. Arch Intern Med 1997;157:57–62.
30 Adams JT, DeWeese JA, Mahoney EB: Intermittent subclavian vein obstruction without thrombolysis. Surgery 1968;63:147–165.
31 Demondion X, Boutry N, Drizenko A, Paul C, Francke JP, Cotten A: Thoracic outlet: anatomic correlation with MR imaging. AJR Am J Roentgenol 2000;175:417–422.
32 Remy-Jardin M, Remy J, Masson P, Bonnel F, Debatselier P, Vinckier L, Duhamel A: Helical CT angiography of thoracic outlet syndrome: functional anatomy. AJR Am J Roentgenol 2000;174:1667–1674.

33 Demondion X, Bacqueville E, Paul C, Duquesnoy B, Hachulla E, Cotten A: Thoracic outlet: assessment with MR imaging in asymptomatic and symptomatic populations. Radiology 2003;227:461–468.
34 Haire WD, Lynch TG, Lund GB, Lieberman RP, Edney JA: Limitations of magnetic resonance imaging and ultrasound-directed (duplex) scanning in the diagnosis of subclavian vein thrombosis. J Vasc Surg 1991;13:391–397.
35 Donayre CE, White GH, Mehringer SM, Wilson SE: Pathogenesis determines late morbidity of axillosubclavian vein thrombosis. Am J Surg 1986;152:179–184.
36 Kammen BF, Soulen MC: Phlegmasia cerulea dolens of the upper extremity. J Vasc Interv Radiol 1995;6:283–286.
37 Harley DP, White RA, Nelson RJ, Mehringer CM: Pulmonary embolism secondary to venous thrombosis of the arm. Am J Surg 1984; 147:221–224.
38 Hicken GJ, Ameli FM: Management of subclavian-axillary vein thrombosis: a review. Can J Surg 1998;41:13–25.
39 Rutherford RB, Hurlbert SN: Primary subclavian-axillary vein thrombosis: consensus and commentary. Cardiovasc Surg 1996;4:420–423.
40 Khan SN, Stansby G: Current management of Paget-Schroetter syndrome in the UK. Ann R Coll Surg Engl 2004;86:29–34.
41 Machleder HI: Evaluation of a new treatment strategy for Paget-Schroetter syndrome: spontaneous thrombosis of the axillary-subclavian vein. J Vasc Surg 1993;17:305–315.
42 Molina JE: Need for emergency treatment in subclavian vein effort thrombosis. J Am Coll Surg 1995;181:414–420.
43 Angle N, Gelabert HA, Farooq MM, Ahn SS, Caswell DR, Freischlag JA, Machleder HI: Safety and efficacy of early surgical decompression of the thoracic outlet for Paget-Schroetter syndrome. Ann Vasc Surg 2001;15:37–42.
44 Lee MC, Grassi CJ, Belkin M, Mannick JA, Whittemore AD, Donaldson MC: Early operative intervention after thrombolytic therapy for primary subclavian vein thrombosis: an effective treatment approach. J Vasc Surg 1998; 27:1101–1107.
45 Lee WA, Hill BB, Harris EJ Jr, Semba CP, Olcott C 4th: Surgical intervention is not required for all patients with subclavian vein thrombosis. J Vasc Surg 2000;32:57–67.
46 Urschel HC Jr, Razzuk MA: Paget-Schroetter syndrome: what is the best management? Ann Thorac Surg 2000;69:1663–1668.
47 Joffe HV, Kucher N, Tapson VF, Goldhaber SZ: Upper-extremity deep vein thrombosis: a prospective registry of 592 patients. Circulation 2004;110:1605–1611.

Acta Hæmatologica

Acta Haematol 2006;115:221–229
DOI: 10.1159/000090939

Exercise-Induced Deep Vein Thrombosis of the Upper Extremity

2. A Case Series in Children

Leonardo R. Brandão[a] Suzan Williams[a] Walter H.A. Kahr[a] Clodagh Ryan[a]
Michael Temple[b] Anthony K.C. Chan[c, d]

[a]Division of Haematology/Oncology, Department of Paediatrics, [b]Department of Diagnostic Imaging, Centre for Image Guided Therapy and [c]Department of Paediatric Laboratory Medicine, The Hospital for Sick Children, Toronto; [d]Department of Paediatrics, McMaster University, Hamilton, Canada

Key Words
Postthrombotic syndrome · Thrombolysis · Upper extremity · Venous thrombosis, effort-related

Abstract
Upper-extremity deep venous thrombosis (UEDVT) is an increasingly important clinical problem in children. These events are classified as primary or secondary, with the latter being the most common and usually associated with the presence of a central venous line. Among primary UEDVT, the so-called Paget-Schroetter syndrome, effort-related or exercise-induced upper-extremity thrombotic event represents an extremely rare finding that has never been described in a pediatric series. The objective of the second part of this two-part article is to report the first pediatric series in a group of adolescents with this condition from a single center, describing their clinical features, management, and outcome. A retrospective chart review of 6 patients seen between December 2003 and April 2005 was conducted, with a median follow-up of 9 months (range 2–17). Four females and two males, all Caucasian, were enrolled with a median age of 16 years (range 14–17). In all cases, strenuous exercise was present in the month preceding diagnosis and mild trauma was present in only one case (weight lifting). At presentation, all patients had objective swelling of the affected limb for a median of 4 days (range 2–14), and 4 patients had UEDVT of the dominant arm. Thrombophilia investigation revealed that 50% had a combined prothrombotic state at presentation, and all patients were/are being treated with anticoagulation for 6 months (low-molecular-weight heparin followed by warfarin). Continuation of the initial symptoms was present in all cases but one at the 3-month clinic follow-up (last case has yet to reach 3 months of follow-up), and residual moderate to severe postthrombotic syndrome was present in all 3 cases followed for more than 12 months. Of those 3 patients followed for more than 1 year, 2 patients recurred despite having complete resolution of the thrombus after 6 months of anticoagulation, and the third patient underwent surgery with clinical improvement. Adolescents with UEDVT treated only with anticoagulation seem to have a poor outcome.

Introduction

Paget-Schroetter syndrome or effort-related thrombosis of the axillary-subclavian vein is a rare but potentially disabling condition that afflicts young healthy individu-

KARGER

Fax +41 61 306 12 34
E-Mail karger@karger.ch
www.karger.com

0001–5792/06/1154–0221$23.50/0

Accessible online at:
www.karger.com/aha

Leonardo R. Brandão, MD
The Hospital for Sick Children, 555 University Avenue, Black Wing, Room 10412
Toronto, Ont. M5G 1X8 (Canada)
Tel. +1 416 813 7500, ext. 5401, Fax +1 416 813 5327
E-Mail leonardo.brandao@sickkids.ca

als, most commonly males. The cause is multifactorial but almost always involves extrinsic compression of the subclavian vein at the thoracic inlet, causing venous stenosis from repetitive trauma. The origin is frequently difficult to define and the clinical presentation ranges from severe discomfort and edema including the forearm and hand, to few or no symptoms at all. Delay in diagnosis and misdiagnoses may prevent prompt therapy, which may contribute to potential complications including thrombosis progression, recurrence, pulmonary embolism, and postphlebitic syndrome. In the earlier section of this article (part 1) [1], we have reviewed the literature in effort-related thrombosis of the axillary-subclavian vein, which is most commonly found in adults. No large prospective studies to access, classify, and describe the natural history of the disease, best methods of diagnosis, and most appropriate treatment have been carried out.

This condition has never been characterized exclusively in children, whose diverse hemostatic system may contribute to a different clinical outcome. In this concluding section (part 2) of this article, the first case series of adolescents diagnosed with this condition is described.

Methods

Study Design

Data collection was done by retrospective chart review performed in a single pediatric institution. Clinical data collected for each patient included the following: age at presentation, ethnicity, gender, body mass index (BMI), underlying medical condition, type and intensity of physical activity, presenting signs and symptoms, upper-extremity deep venous thrombosis (UEDVT) location and radiologic findings, acquired and inherited thrombophilia results, type and intensity of anticoagulation regimen, and clinical outcome. Family history of thrombosis, defined as a first- and/or second-degree relative with venous thromboembolism (VTEs), was recorded.

Patient Population

The study population consisted of nonselected, consecutive children diagnosed with effort-related UEDVT confirmed by imaging methods from December 2003 to May 2005. The patients enrolled were being followed by the Thrombosis Program at The Hospital for Sick Children (Sick Kids) in Toronto, Canada.

Radiologic and Vascular Investigation

In the study center, ultrasonography was used to detect UEDVT. Ultrasonography was performed utilizing a high-resolution real-time scanner equipped with 5- to 12-MHz linear array transducers and by applying compression to the venous territory. With compression ultrasonography, UEDVT was diagnosed when compressibility in the transverse and longitudinal planes failed to occlude the lumen of the affected vein. When compression could not be performed due to its location, the finding of focal intraluminal filling defect, the absence of a color signal, or change of flow detected by color Doppler ultrasonography confirmed clinical suspicion of UEDVT. All patients were submitted to bilateral upper extremity compression Doppler ultrasonography and unilateral venography. Regarding venograms, patients were studied with the examined arm in extension (6 patients) and abducted to 90° (4 patients). A nonionic contrast (Omnipaque 300®) was injected in both arms, and to avoid preferential filling, pressure was applied to the cervical veins. Thrombosis was excluded if the entire deep venous system of the arm was visualized and if it was free from intraluminal defects. Plain chest films and/or chest computerized tomography was utilized in all patients to rule out a cervical rib or other anatomic abnormalities. Patients with a suspicion of thoracic outlet syndrome (TOS) were also submitted to pulse volume recording and arterial duplex ultrasound testing. This noninvasive test allows a qualitative, reproducible assessment of pulse volume recording in arteries in two different points of the upper limb (proximal and distal), generating a rapid upstroke and downstroke pulse with narrow complex in cases of normal arterial flow. In cases of structural and/or functional obstruction of the affected arm with provocative maneuvers, abnormal pulses are found, allowing the delimitation of the arm area with potential vessel compression [2].

Laboratory Analysis

All children diagnosed with an UEDVT at HSC were investigated for an acquired and an inherited prothrombotic condition either at diagnosis before therapy was commenced, at the end of anticoagulation treatment, or during their clinical follow-up visits provided that the investigation had not been completed previously. For this study, abnormal plasma-based results that might have been affected acutely by the VTE were considered inconclusive. All assay results were compared with previously generated age-appropriate values [3, 4]. Thrombophilia testing included collection for antithrombin (AT), protein C, free protein S, factor V (FV) Leiden, prothrombin G20210A and methylenetetrahydrofolate reductase (MTHFR) C677T mutation, activated protein C resistance, anticardiolipin antibody, and lupus anticoagulant (LA). The protocol for sample collection and processing, as well as data interpretation has been reported in a previous publication [5]. Factor VIII (FVIII) level, factor IX (FIX) level, and factor XI (FXI) level were measured by a standard one-stage clotting assay. Elevated FVIII, FIX and FXI levels were defined as levels above the 97.5th percentile from age-matched controls [3, 4]. Plasma lipoprotein (a) [Lp(a)] was measured with an ELISA (Trinity Biotech, Jamestown, N.Y., USA), and homocysteine levels were measured by tandem mass spectrometry (Micromass, Quatro Ultima Mass Spectometer, UK).

Anticoagulation Therapy

In accordance to the hospital protocol for effort-related UEDVT that is under development, children with this condition should receive at least 6 months of full-dose anticoagulation therapy. Anticoagulation therapy would be initiated with low-molecular-weight heparin (LMWH), followed by oral anticoagulation with warfarin to keep an international normalized ratio (INR) between 2.0 and 3.0.

Follow-Up Protocol and Outcome

Patients diagnosed with this condition were scheduled to be seen in clinic after 3, 6 and 12 months from the initial event with subsequent clinic visits every year. Recurrence of UEDVT was based on new clinical findings confirmed by radiologic examination. The diagnosis of postthrombotic syndrome (PTS) and their follow-up was based on the application of a standardized pediatric PTS score previously published [6]. This pediatric scale adapted from an adult scale [7] has been applied in a previous cross-sectional study evaluating PTS in children [6]. The scale was applied to the upper extremity involved, and it included the following information: (1) subjective symptoms (n = 2), reported by the patient, with results registered as absent (score = 0) or present (score = 1) and (2) objective signs (n = 9), which were graded similarly (Appendix). The items varicosities and edema of the head were graded on a 3-point Likert scale (absent = 0, moderate = 1, severe = 2). The presence of ulceration automatically classified the patient's score as severe. All signs and symptoms were added with a maximum score of 12. The classification of PTS was listed as mild (score = 1–3), moderate (score = 4–8), or severe (score >8 or presence of ulceration).

Table 1. Patient description

Patient	Sex/age years	BMI kg/m^2	Location/ dominant arm	Delay to onset, days	Sport
1	F/15	21.8	R subclavian/yes	7	rowing
2	F/17	21.8	L subclavian/no	3	swimming
3	F/16	18.6	L subclavian/yes	4	dancing
4	M/17	26.6[a]	L subclavian/no	2	swimming
5	M/16	22.6	R axillary/yes	14	weight lifting
6	F/14	20.1	R axillary/yes	2	dancing

R = Right; L = left.
[a] Patient is very bulky.

Results

Epidemiology

From December 2003 to May 2005, 6 consecutive children with effort-related UEDVT were followed in the Thrombosis Clinic at Sick Kids. Two males and 4 females, all Caucasian and aged between 14 and 17 years (median age 16 years), have been followed for a median of 9 months (range 2–17 months). In addition, all patients were healthy, and only 1 patient had a minor trauma to his elbow prior to the initial onset of his UEDVT (patient 5; table 1). None of the patients had a central venous line (CVL) placed in the past, a previous recent infection, surgery to the affected limb, or any other vascular and/or anatomic malformation. None of the females were using or had used oral contraception, and none of the patients had diabetes, hypertension and/or exposure to tobacco, alcohol, or performance-enhancing drugs.

In all cases, strenuous exercise (2 dancing, 1 competitive rowing, 2 competitive swimming, 1 weight lifting) was present in the month or week preceding the diagnosis (table 1). All patients were involved in physical training for at least 12 h per week and both swimmers had 2-hour sessions twice per day. All patients had a history of recent escalation of their already intense physical activity schedule in the week preceding the diagnosis of VTE. In 4 cases, the dominant arm was the upper limb involved. With the exception of 1 patient, all patients had a BMI between 18.5 and 24.9, which is encountered in normal nonobese people. The single patient with a BMI between 25.0 and 29.9 (26.6), which is usually reflective of obesity, was in actuality an extremely muscular person.

Clinical Signs and Symptoms

At presentation, all patients had objective swelling of the affected limb for a median of 4 days (range 2–14), 5 had arm color changes (1 with paleness, 4 with bluish color that improved with arm rest), 4 had a sensation of fullness, and 2 had intermittent paresthesia (table 2). No patients had an abnormal sensation or pain of their 4th or 5th finger ipsilateral to the UEDVT, which can be related to injury of the brachial plexus.

During the first physical examination done at Sick Kids, all patients were subjected to the same provocative maneuvers for assessment of TOS. These maneuvers were applied by one of the three physicians from the Thrombosis Service at Sick Kids. They consisted of either extending the patient's arm on the affected side while the patient extends the neck and rotates the head toward the same side (Adson's test) or abducting and externally rotating the same arm with UEDVT (Wright's test). On both tests, weakening of the ipsilateral radial pulse suggests compression of the subclavian artery. At presentation no patient had positive provocative maneuver results, although 1 patient presented with intermittent arm discoloration that resolved spontaneously. Palpation of the supraclavicular region for detection of brachial plexus tenderness or masses was noncontributory in all cases. None of the patients had pitting edema or clinical findings suggestive of phlegmasia cerulea dolens.

Imaging Findings

Initially, all patients had bilateral Doppler compressive ultrasound. Radiologic findings identified 4 subclavian vein thrombosis and 2 axillary vein thrombosis (1 axillary vein alone and 1 combined axillary/subclavian veins), with 5 cases being nonocclusive at presentation

Table 2. Patient presentation and follow-up

Patient	Initial findings	Initial imaging: (occl. vs. non-occl.)	PTS score at 3 months; Δ arm circ.	PTS score at 6 months; Δ arm circ.	PTS score at 12 months; Δ arm circ.
1	F	non-occl.	5; 2 cm	6; 2.6 cm	7[a]; 2.5 cm
2	F, S, C, P, PR	non-occl.	n/a	n/a	n/a
3	F, S, C	non-occl.	5; 1 cm	n/a	n/a
4	F, S, C	non-occl.	4; 2 cm	n/a	n/a
5	F, S, C	non-occl.	5; 1.5 cm	6; 2.5 cm[b]	7; 3.5 cm
6	S, C, P, PR	occl.	5; 1.5 cm	6; 2.5 cm[c]	6–7; 2.5 cm

occl. = Occlusive; non-occl. = nonocclusive; Δ arm circ. = difference of arm circumference; S = swelling; F = fullness; C = color change; P = pain; PR = paresthesia; n/a = not available.

[a] Even though score represents moderate PTS, unable to utilize arm for minimal functions, such as writing.

[b] UEDVT recurred 3 weeks after discontinuation of 6-month anticoagulation therapy despite previous objective thrombus resolution.

[c] UEDVT recurred 3 months after discontinuation of 6-month anticoagulation therapy.

Table 3. Thrombophilia panel results

Patient	FV Leiden	PT G20210A	MTHFR	HCY μmol/l	Lp(a) mg/dl	APCR	PC IU/ml	PS IU/ml
1	–	–	n/a	3.8	9.9	2.3	1.06	0.88
2	–	–	n/a	n/a	n/a	n/a	0.84	0.8
3	–	–	homoz.[a]	5.7	11.8	n/a	n/a	n/a
4	homoz.[a]	–	heteroz.	5.7	7.1	1.3[a]	n/a	n/a
5	heteroz.[a]	–	heteroz.	6	5.5	1.8[a]	0.71	1.19
6	–	–	n/a	6.7	17.1	n/a	0.91	0.56

PT G20210A = Prothrombin G20210A mutation; MTHFR = methylenetetrahydrofolate reductase mutation; HCY = homocysteine; Lp(a) = lipoprotein (a); APCR = activated protein C resistance; PC = protein C; PS = protein S; – = negative; n/a = not available; homoz. = homozygous; heteroz. = heterozygous.

[a] Results represent abnormal values.

and with 4 UEDVT occurring in the dominant arm. Further imaging, including unilateral venographies in all patients and a plain chest X-ray (5 patients) and/or chest computerized tomography (4 patients) excluded vascular malformations or anatomic abnormalities in all patients. The arterial duplex ultrasound was done in 3 patients, being suggestive of TOS in all cases.

Inherited or Acquired Thrombophilia Conditions

Three patients presented with normal results and the 3 others with combined abnormalities. In the group of patients with normal results, 1 had a complete normal panel, 1 awaits the results for AT, FVIII, FIX, FXI levels and Lp(a) with the rest of the panel being normal, and the third patient had a transiently positive LA. In the group of patients with combined abnormalities, the first presented with combined homozygous MTHFR (but with normal fasting homocysteine level) and an elevated FVIII level (2.50 IU/ml) at presentation that will be repeated at the end of therapy. The other 2 patients' abnormal findings were as follows: (1) 1 with homozygous FV Leiden and transiently elevated FVIII level (1.88 IU/ml) and (2) 1 with heterozygous FV Leiden, and transiently elevated FVIII level (1.85 IU/ml) and positive LA (tables 3, 4). Overall, a positive family history was found in 3 patients, including 1 patient with a first-degree cousin with lower

Table 4. Thrombophilia panel results

Patient	AT IU/ml	LAC	ACA	FVIII IU/ml	FIX IU/ml	FXI IU/ml
1	1.2	–	–	1.14	0.47	0.93
2	n/a	–	borderline	n/a	n/a	n/a
3	1.06	–	–	2.5[a]	0.57	n/a
4	1.05	–	–	1.88[a]	0.54	1.05
5	0.89	pos.[a]; –	–	1.85[a]; 1.07	0.85	1.04
6	1.13	pos.[a]; –	–	1.28	1.1	1.3

AT = Antithrombin; LAC = lupus anticoagulant; ACA = anticardiolipin antibody; – = negative; n/a = nonavailable; pos. = positive.
[a] Results represent abnormal values.

extremity deep vein thrombosis (DVT) at the age of 37 years, a second patient with a maternal grandmother that developed lower-extremity DVT in her 50s, and a third patient whose maternal grandmother is on long-term oral anticoagulation (unknown reason).

Anticoagulation Therapy

In all cases, anticoagulation therapy was started with LMWH (enoxaparin in 2 patients, dalteparin in 2 and tinzaparin in the remaining 2). All patients were also started on oral anticoagulation (warfarin) within 1 week of therapy to keep the INR between 2.0 and 3.0. The anticoagulant doses of both LMWH and warfarin were calculated according to the pediatric recommendations of the Seventh American College of Chest Physicians Conference (ACCP) on Antithrombotic and Thrombolytic Therapy [8]. All patients were compliant to their treatment, and their anticoagulant monitoring (INR or anti-Xa) was within the therapeutic range during their entire anticoagulation therapy.

Follow-Up and Outcome

Half of the patients were followed for more than 12 months. In 2 of these 3 patients, VTE recurrence occurred 3 weeks and 3 months after discontinuation of oral anticoagulation (patients 5 and 6, respectively; tables 1, 2). In the first case, thrombus resolution was documented by ultrasonography 3 months after initiation of therapy, and treatment was continued for a total of 6 months. Venous thromboembolic event recurrence occurred with an occlusive thrombus, now present in the right brachiocephalic vein detected initially by ultrasound and confirmed by CT venogram. In the second case, no residual thrombus was present by ultrasonography at 3 months and treatment was given for a total of 6 months. Recurrence involved the same vessel location with an occlusive VTE confirmed by ultrasonography 3 months after cessation of oral anticoagulation. This patient is scheduled for surgery after confirmation of TOS done by clinical assessment and by arterial duplex ultrasound. In both cases the patients were previously stable, presenting with acute onset of new subjective and objective findings. Also in both cases, the initial thrombus was present in the axillary vein, where clot resolution was documented by normal compression but not by a venogram. The third patient of this group was submitted to catheter-guided fibrinolysis followed by first rib resection after she presented with major arm function impairment accompanied by TOS. The protocol for fibrinolysis that was utilized prior to surgery has been previously published [9]. Multisidehole infusion catheter containing urokinase (120,000–180,000 IU/h) was inserted, and success of thrombolysis was assessed by serial venograms at 6- to 12-hour intervals.

No minor or major bleeding episodes occurred in any patient, and no one received local and/or systemic fibrinolysis at the time of initial presentation.

In regard to PTS, 3 patients were followed for more than 12 months. In those 3 patients there was subjective and objective progression of PTS, such as the inability to write in patient 1 and pain requiring control with amytriptiline in patient 6 (tables 3, 4). More specifically, PTS scores progressed from 5 to 7 in 2 of the patients followed for more than 1 year, and from 5 to 8 in the third patient. All patients from this study were oriented to use custom-made graduate compression Jobst stockings on the affected arm with 30 mm Hg compression after the first month of diagnosis.

Of the 3 patients found to have TOS, 1 patient has not completed 6 months of follow-up, currently continuing on anticoagulation. The other 2 patients were followed for at least 1 year, having either recurred or presented with severe PTS that warranted surgical decompression.

Discussion

Although the clinical significance of primary effort-related subclavian-axillary thrombosis has been increasingly recognized in the past years, this entity has not been characterized in children. We report for the first time a series of patients with Paget-Schroetter syndrome or effort-related UEDVT which includes only patients within the pediatric age range (adolescents). This first report shows that in children, this entity may have a worse clinical progression and outcome compared to adults. Unlike CVL-induced UEDVT in children, where many cases are asymptomatic, all of our patients presented with pronounced symptoms which included swelling without pitting edema, color changes, pain, and paresthesia. The initial symptoms persisted at the initial 3-month follow-up for all patients (the most recent has yet to complete 3 months post-diagnosis), and were still present for the 3 patients followed longest, all of whom developed PTS. In effort-related UEDVT in children, a positive correlation between persistence of symptoms and the development of PTS is suggested by the preliminary findings of this series. In all patients symptoms were exacerbated by minor physical activities or weight bearing with the affected arm (e.g. carrying a backpack).

Recurrence occurred in 2 patients whose previous imaging findings had objectively documented thrombus resolution by ultrasound. An important point raised is to question if clot resolution should in fact be documented by the 'gold standard' venography rather than by the former method, and if in those 2 cases the documentation of thrombus resolution obtained by ultrasound was in fact an inadequate reflection of a residual clot in the presence of an aggravated PTS. Obtaining a venogram at the end of therapy would also contribute to a better delineation of the incidence of clot recurrence and of PTS in this condition in children.

The 2 VTE recurrences occurred shortly after discontinuation of warfarin (3 weeks to 3 months) in the ipsilateral arm involved, but in only 1 patient was TOS documented. TOS is an important confounder in the analysis of our data, given that the 2 patients diagnosed with TOS that were followed for more than 12 months have either recurred (1 patient) or underwent surgery due to symptom progression (1 patient).

The thrombophilia investigation of the 2 patients with recurrence showed one patient heterozygous for FV Leiden and transiently elevated FVIII and LA, and another with a transient LA. The other patient with homozygosity for FV Leiden has not yet completed 6 months of follow-up. The role of acquired and inherited thrombotic conditions in the outcome of effort-related and non-CVL-related UEDVT remains unanswered.

There are very few publications on the prevalence of acquired or inherited thrombophilia in primary UEDVT [10]. While adult patients diagnosed with primary UEDVT and thrombophilia seem to have a higher rate of thrombosis recurrence [11], the contribution of thrombophilic states to effort-related UEDVT in adult patients seems to be less than to idiopathic UEDVT [10, 12]. Differently from these findings, our case series has shown a high incidence of combined thrombophilia, which may reflect the necessity of their presence to counterbalance the lower baseline thrombin generation found in children [13]. In adolescents, a more aggressive behavior of this condition may be a consequence of their physiological decreased fibrinolysis [14], even though endurance exercise training seems to improve fibrinolysis in normal subjects [15]. In summary, the role of inherited or acquired thrombophilia in the development of an unfavorable outcome needs to be clarified in a larger pediatric series with this condition.

In terms of management and outcome, our findings were again surprising. All patients were uniformly treated with 'classic' anticoagulation consisting of LMWH followed by warfarin. Despite the small number of patients reported and the relatively short clinical follow-up, a considerable percentage of patients have already presented with poor clinical outcomes, as defined by UEDVT recurrence, the presence of PTS or the necessity of surgery. Of the 3 patients followed for more than 12 months, 2 had VTE recurrence and the other underwent thrombolysis immediately followed by first rib resection because of significant symptoms.

The outcome in this study may even be worse than what the PTS scores suggest. While no patient had a PTS score above 8 (= moderate), the score was not entirely reflective of some patients' clinical status. Within the group followed for more than 12 months, 2 patients progressively presented with arm function impairment not reflected by the scale used (e.g. the same score 1 for pain or abnormal arm use from the PTS scale was given regardless of amount of limb function impairment). The level of impairment encountered in our patients was progressive, initially presenting as pain or discomfort of the affected arm with aerobic activities, followed by the same complaints with regular activities, and by complaints at rest. The advantage of the scale utilized here is its easy applicability, allowing a quick assessment of patients of a younger age that would otherwise probably not be able to provide detailed information. However, some clinical data may be lost in the use of the current scale. Likewise, because of the lack of a 'gold standard' objective validated clinical scale to diagnose PTS and quantify its severity in the upper extremity of adults and children, an adaptation may be necessary to improve the evaluation of PTS in the upper limb.

In the initial publications on effort-related UEDVT, persistent symptoms were present in 20% of cases, and the comparison of different treatment modalities favored anticoagulation over rest and elevation [16]. Later reports have registered 75% of patients with some type of residual disability at an average of 6.6 years [17]. A specific analysis of PTS functional disability and quality of life (QOL) in 24 adult patients was recently reported [18]. At a median assessment time of 13 months, daily ipsilateral arm or hand swelling was present in 52% of patients, and arm pain in 20% of patients. In comparison to the patients without PTS, patients with UEDVT and PTS had significantly more function disability (calculated by specific arm DASH score, mean value 20.9 vs. 3.7; $p = 0.009$) and poorer QOL (calculated by VEINES-QOL score, mean value 45.6 vs. 53.6; $p = 0.001$). Patients with dominant arm PTS appear to do worse than those with non-dominant arm PTS. These results of persistent symptoms and functional impairment corroborate our findings of increased morbidity after UEDVT in a relatively short period of time despite adequate anticoagulant treatment.

A perhaps similar group of patients in comparison to our series was described by Arko et al. [19], who reported 26 high-performance athletes aged between 17 and 40 years diagnosed with VTE of the subclavian vein, axillary/subclavian artery, popliteal artery, or iliac artery. Twelve cases (46% of the total) had effort-related UEDVT, with a mean age of 23.3 years (range 16–25 years). All patients from this subgroup received thrombolytic therapy, with total clot lysis in 8 patients and partial success (<50% clot reduction) in the remaining 4 patients. The latter were patients that underwent lysis after 4 weeks of 'classic' anticoagulation. Eight patients underwent TOS decompression surgically without significant morbidity. All 8 patients had a resolution of their presenting symptoms, with an average follow-up of 13.9 months (range 4–26 months). The 4 remaining patients of this subgroup treated with 'classic' anticoagulation after initial fibrinolysis also had minimal symptoms at the end of their anticoagulant therapy (average 3.6 months). This group of athletic patients seemed to have a better outcome than our patients, despite having surgery or oral anticoagulation. The difference of this series in comparison to ours is that all patients from this study were initially treated with fibrinolytic therapy, raising the question about its role in the prevention of long-term UEDVT complications.

Because of the increasing rate of complications reported in the most recent series in patients with this condition, there has been a trend towards interventional procedures in the management of effort-related UEDVT. Furthermore, the advocates of this strategy defend that prompt removal of the thrombus is associated with decreased long-term complications, even though this statement is not based on randomized clinic studies. A non-randomized study comparing the use of oral anticoagulation and thrombolysis in adults with subclavian-axillary VTE included 95 patients [20]. Thrombolysis was applied in 33 individuals, with a success rate of 88% and a bleeding complication rate of 21%. No bleeding was observed in any patient treated conservatively. Even though there was a 60% risk reduction of residual subclavian thrombus in the group treated with oral medication, there was no difference of symptomatic PTS among both groups. An American consensus obtained from 25 vascular surgeons highlighted some of the current trends in treating this entity [21]. Seventy percent of the participants felt it was appropriate to intervene (thrombectomy or thrombolysis), especially in those who needed to restart their physical activity soon. Ninety-six percent felt the most indicated intervention was catheter-guided thrombolysis therapy, defining 2 weeks as a limit of effective thrombolytic therapy. A similar consensus that specifically discussed effort-related UEDVT was held in the UK in 2004 [22]. Thrombolysis was once more the most common treatment modality among surgeons (86.7%). Stenting was not an option entertained due to its high rate of complications. The most striking finding was the lack of consensus regarding the type of procedure, timing of the surgery, and surgical approach for management of UEDVT.

In pediatrics, there have been no studies reporting the outcome of this entity alone, but there are several reports of the overall incidence of PTS, ranging from 7 to 70% after 2–5 years of follow-up [6, 23–31]. Manco-Johnson and colleagues [31] have recently found a higher incidence of PTS, residual thrombus, or VTE recurrence with an elevated FVIII level and D-dimers. Interestingly, 1 patient from our series that recurred and that had PTS presented with a high FVIII level that normalized after 6 months.

Revel-Vilk et al. [32] suggested arterial location and nonocclusive thrombus as the only predictors of an increased thrombus resolution rate, whereas lack of VTE resolution by radiographic assessment, number of vessels involved in the initial VTE, and length of follow-up were proposed by Kuhle et al. [6] as risk factors for PTS development. In adults, the development of PTS correlates to ipsilateral VTE recurrence and high BMI [33, 34]. Regarding effort-related UEDVT, high BMI may not be a factor influencing outcome, since the patients involved are usually healthy and fit.

Conclusion

Our series showed that adolescents diagnosed with exercise-induced UEDVT treated with anticoagulant alone have a poor outcome. Whether or not the use of a more aggressive approach such as thrombolytic therapy can improve outcome requires more support. A larger number of children with this entity needs to be followed to help answering some of the questions raised by our findings.

Acknowledgments

We wish to thank Dr. Fred Pluthero and Ms. Lu Ann Brooker for the critical review of the manuscript. Anthony K.C. Chan is a recipient of a Career Investigator Award from the Heart and Stroke Foundation of Canada.

Appendix. Post-phlebitic syndrome questionnaire

Post-Phlebitic Syndrome Scoring Sheet			Name: ....
Height:	Weight:	Dominant side:	ID: ....
Location of Thrombus:			Age: ....
Date of Thrombosis:			DOB: ....
CVL-related:	☐ Yes	☐ No	Date: ....

SUBJECTIVE	ABSENT (Score: 0)	PRESENT (Score: 1)	N/A
Pain or abnormal use	☐	☐	☐
Swelling	☐	☐	☐

OBJECTIVE	ABSENT (Score: 0)	PRESENT (Score: 1)	N/A
Change in skin color	☐	☐	☐
Limb circumference increased	☐	☐	☐
Pitting edema	☐	☐	☐
Collaterals in the skin	☐	☐	☐
Pigmentation	☐	☐	☐
Tenderness on palpation	☐	☐	☐

OBJECTIVE	ABSENT (Score: 0)	MODERATE (Score: 1)	SEVERE (Score: 2)	N/A
Edema of the head	☐	☐	☐	☐
Varicosities	☐	☐	☐	☐
Ulcerations	☐	☐	☐	☐

MEASUREMENTS (cm)	LEFT	RIGHT DIFFERENCE	N/A
Upper arm			☐
Thigh			☐
Calf			☐

References

1 Brandão LR, Williams S, Kahr WHA, Ryan C, Temple M, Chan AKC: Exercise-induced deep vein thrombosis of the upper extremity. 1. Literature review. Acta Haematol 2006;115:214–220.

2 Baxter BT, Blackburn D, Payne K, Pearce WH, Yao JS: Noninvasive evaluation of the upper extremity. Surg Clin North Am 1990;70/1:87–97.

3 Goodnight SH Jr, Hathaway W: Disorders of Hemostasis and Thrombosis – A Clinical Guide. New York, McGraw-Hill, 2001.

4 Andrew M, Monagle P, Brooker L: Thromboembolic Complications during Infancy and Childhood. Hamilton, BC Decker, 2000.

5 deVeber G, Monagle P, Chan A, MacGregor D, Curtis R, Lee S, Vegh P, Adams M, Marzinotto V, Leaker M, Massicotte MP, Lillicrap D, Andrew M: Prothrombotic disorders in infants and children with cerebral thromboembolism. Arch Neurol 1998;55:1539–1543.

6 Kuhle S, Koloshuk B, Marzinotto V, Bauman M, Massicotte P, Andrew M, Chan A, Abdolell M, Mitchell L: A cross-sectional study evaluating post-thrombotic syndrome in children. Thromb Res 2003;111/4–5:227–233.

7 Villalta S, Bagatella P, Piccioli A: Assessment of validity and reproducibility of a clinical scale for the post-thrombotic syndrome (abstract). Haemostasis 1994;24:158a.

8 Monagle P, Chan A, Massicotte P, Chalmers E, Michelson AD: Antithrombotic therapy in children: the Seventh ACCP Conference on Antithrombotic and Thrombolytic Therapy. Chest 2004;126(3 suppl):645S–687S.

9 Harley DP, White RA, Nelson RJ, Mehringer CM: Pulmonary embolism secondary to venous thrombosis of the arm. Am J Surg 1984; 147/2:221–224.

10 Heron E, Lozinguez O, Alhenc-Gelas M, Emmerich J, Fiessinger JN: Hypercoagulable states in primary upper-extremity deep vein thrombosis. Arch Intern Med 2000;160:382–386.

11 Martinelli I, Battaglioli T, Bucciarelli P, Passamonti SM, Mannucci PM: Risk factors and recurrence rate of primary deep vein thrombosis of the upper extremities. Circulation 2004; 110:566–570.

12 Hendler MF, Meschengieser SS, Blanco AN, Alberto MF, Salviu MJ, Gennari L, Lazzari MA: Primary upper-extremity deep vein thrombosis: high prevalence of thrombophilic defects. Am J Hematol 2004;76:330–337.

13 Andrew M, Mitchell L, Vegh P, Ofosu F: Thrombin regulation in children differs from adults in the absence and presence of heparin. Thromb Haemost 1994;72:836–842.

14 Siegbahn A, Ruusuvaara L: Age dependence of blood fibrinolytic components and the effects of low-dose oral contraceptives on coagulation and fibrinolysis in teenagers. Thromb Haemost 1988;60:361–364.

15 Killewich LA, Macko RF, Montgomery PS, Wiley LA, Gardner AW: Exercise training enhances endogenous fibrinolysis in peripheral arterial disease. J Vasc Surg 2004;40:741–745.

16 Hughes ES: Venous obstruction in upper extremity (Paget-Schroetter's syndrome). Review of 320 cases. Int Abstr Surg 1949;88:89–127.

17 Tilney ML, Griffiths HJ, Edwards EA: Natural history of major venous thrombosis of the upper extremity. Arch Surg 1970;101:792–796.

18 Kahn SR, Elman EA, Bornais C, Blostein M, Wells PS: Post-thrombotic syndrome, functional disability and quality of life after upper extremity deep venous thrombosis in adults. Thromb Haemost 2005;93:499–502.

19 Arko FR, Harris EJ, Zarins CK, Olcott C: Vascular complications in high-performance athletes. J Vasc Surg 2001;33:935–942.

20 Sabeti S, Schillinger M, Mlekusch W, Haumer M, Ahmadi R, Minar E: Treatment of subclavian-axillary vein thrombosis: long-term outcome of anticoagulation versus systemic thrombolysis. Thromb Res 2002;108/5–6: 279–285.

21 Rutherford RB, Hurlbert SN: Primary subclavian-axillary vein thrombosis: consensus and commentary. Cardiovasc Surg 1996;4:420–423.

22 Khan SN, Stansby G: Current management of Paget-Schroetter syndrome in the UK. Ann R Coll Surg Engl 2004;86/1:29–34.

23 Andrew M, David M, Adams M, Ali K, Anderson R, Barnard D, Bernstein M, Brisson L, Cairney B, DeSai D: Venous thromboembolic complications (VTE) in children: first analyses of the Canadian Registry of VTE. Blood 1994; 83:1251–1257.

24 Gorenstein A, Katz S, Levy P, Schiller M: Noniatrogenic deep vein thrombosis of lower extremities in children. Z Kinderchir 1986;41: 375–378.

25 Massicotte MP, Dix D, Monagle P, Adams M, Andrew M: Central venous catheter related thrombosis in children: analysis of the Canadian Registry of Venous Thromboembolic Complications. J Pediatr 1998;133:770–776.

26 Monagle P, Adams M, Mahoney M, Ali K, Barnard D, Bernstein M, Brisson L, David M, Desai S, Scully MF, Halton J, Israels S, Jardine L, Leaker M, McCusker P, Silva M, Wu J, Anderson R, Andrew M, Massicotte MP: Outcome of pediatric thromboembolic disease: a report from the Canadian Childhood Thrombophilia Registry. Pediatr Res 2000;47:763–766.

27 Hausler M, Hubner D, Delhaas T, Muhler EG: Long term complications of inferior vena cava thrombosis. Arch Dis Child 2001;85/3:228–233.

28 Gurgey A, Aslan D: Outcome of noncatheter-related thrombosis in children: influence of underlying or coexisting factors. J Pediatr Hematol Oncol 2001;23/3:159–164.

29 Marzinotto V, Choi M, Massicotte MP: Post-thrombotic syndrome in children with previous deep vein thrombosis (abstract). Thromb Haemost 2001;78(suppl):OC962.

30 van Ommen CH, Ottenkamp J, Lam J, Brennickmeier M, Heijmans HS, Buller HR, Peters M: The risk of postthrombotic syndrome in children with congenital heart disease. J Pediatr 2002;141:582–586.

31 Goldenberg NA, Knapp-Clevenger R, Manco-Johnson MJ: Elevated plasma factor VIII and D-dimer levels as predictors of poor outcomes of thrombosis in children. N Engl J Med 2004; 351:1081–1088.

32 Revel-Vilk S, Sharathkumar A, Massicotte P, Marzinotto V, Daneman A, Dix D, Chan A: Natural history of arterial and venous thrombosis in children treated with low molecular weight heparin: a longitudinal study by ultrasound. J Thromb Haemost 2004;2/1:42–46.

33 Prandoni P, Villalta S, Bagatella P, Rossi L, Marchiori A, Piccioli A, Bernardi E, Girolami B, Simioni P, Girolami A: The clinical course of deep-vein thrombosis. Prospective long-term follow-up of 528 symptomatic patients. Haematologica 1997;82:423–428.

34 Ageno W, Piantanida E, Dentali F, Steidl L, Mera V, Squizzato A, Marchesi C, Venco A: Body mass index is associated with the development of the post-thrombotic syndrome. Thromb Haemost 2003;89:305–309.

Acta Hæmatologica

Acta Haematol 2006;115:230–236
DOI: 10.1159/000090940

Long-Term Treatment of Thrombosis with Enoxaparin in Pediatric and Adolescent Patients

Nick Merkel[a] Gudrun Günther[b] Rosemarie Schobess[a]

[a] Universitätsklinik und Poliklinik für Kinder- und Jugendmedizin, Martin-Luther-Universität Halle-Wittenberg, Halle/Saale, und [b] Universitätsklinik und Poliklinik für Kinder- und Jugendmedizin, Otto-von-Guericke-Universität, Magdeburg, Deutschland

Key Words

Enoxaparin · Thrombosis · Pediatric · Long-term treatment

Abstract

Thrombosis is a rare event in childhood and adolescence. Nevertheless, increasing numbers of invasive diagnostic and therapeutic procedures also result in increasing numbers of thromboses in pediatric cases, necessitating effective antithrombotic treatment regimens. In recent years, low-molecular-weight heparins (LMWH) in particular have been proved to be a safe and effective alternative to unfractioned heparins. However, the application of LMWH in pediatric patients has not been supported by a single controlled study so far. Furthermore, there is no official approval of these drugs for children. In this pilot study 27 children with deep venous thromboses (DVT) were treated with the LMWH enoxaparin at a dosage of 1.5 mg/kg body weight b.i.d. in neonates and infants and 1 mg/kg body weight b.i.d. in children. This dosage was lowered for prophylaxis if therapeutic success was achieved. The aim of the study was to investigate both, efficacy with respect to patency rates and safety during acute and long-term follow-up. Sufficient therapeutic success required a rapid production of anti-Xa target activity and was reached in 85% of the treated patients, who showed patency of the affected vessel at last follow-up. The mean duration of treatment with full dosage was 16.5 days, followed by prophylaxis over a mean duration of 9.8 months. Rethrombosis or adverse events including heparin-induced thrombocytopenia were not observed in any patient. In conclusion, enoxaparin provides an effective and safe alternative to unfractioned heparins in the treatment of thrombosis in infancy, childhood and adolescence.

Introduction

Venous and arterial vascular occlusions in children are rare with a total incidence of 0.07 events per 10,000 children below the age of 16 years. They spontaneously occur mainly in newborns. A second peak can be observed before and during puberty [1, 2, 6].

Due to an increasing number of invasive interventions in children, such as cardiac catheters, umbilical vessel catheterizations, the application of central venous indwelling systems and not least improved diagnostics, 'thrombosis' may be diagnosed with a higher frequency and at an earlier stage. In many centers, the total number of cases clearly increased over the last 10 years. This urgently necessitates a reevaluation of the actual incidence [5, 7, 8, 16].

KARGER

Fax +41 61 306 12 34
E-Mail karger@karger.ch
www.karger.com

0001–5792/06/1154–0230$23.50/0

Accessible online at:
www.karger.com/aha

Rosemarie Schobess, MD
University Children's Hospital Halle/Saale
Ernst-Grube-Strasse 40, DE–06120 Halle/Saale (Germany)
Tel. +49 345 557 2493, Fax +49 345 557 2843
E-Mail rosemarie.schobess@medizin.uni-halle.de

Nicotine consumption, surgical interventions, immobilization, trauma, lipometabolic disorders, oral contraception, dehydration, sepsis, autoimmune, perinatal and oncologic diseases are exogenous trigger factors [3, 4, 12, 16, 21, 35]. However, there is also a group of endogenous factors, namely hereditary dispositions, the number of which is steadily increasing [10, 11, 13].

Whereas renal vein and sinus vein thrombosis (SVT) show a higher incidence during the neonatal period, thrombosis occurrence shifts during puberty into the distribution pattern observed in adults [6, 13, 14, 51, 52]. The deep venous thrombosis (DVT) predominates. Ninety percent involve the lower half of the body [54]. Symptomatic catheter-associated thrombosis, mainly connected to an increasing number of interventions in the fields of cardiology, oncology and intensive care, are equally spread throughout all the age groups [5, 7, 8, 16].

There are several options for the treatment of thromboses in childhood. However, hitherto no controlled study on the treatment of thrombosis in children has been done. Worldwide, pediatric patients are treated according to adapted recommendations originally made for adults. A separate approval of antithrombotic drugs for children, such as heparins or vitamin K antagonists, currently does not exist. Active thrombolytic therapy and surgical intervention are indicated in cases of acute thromboses or if there is a threat of the loss of organs or extremities. A relative indication is given in cases of catheter-associated occlusion where placement directly on the clot is possible [50, 55, 56].

Another treatment option are heparins. For a long time, unfractioned heparins have been the first choice for treatment of thrombosis during childhood. However, over the last years therapy using low-molecular-weight heparins (LMWH) has increasingly gained importance. This notwithstanding only a few small studies on treatment with LMWH in children have been conducted, almost all of which are limited to therapy in the acute phase [26–33, 36, 37, 49].

We, therefore, conducted this pilot study on the treatment of thrombosis in children following the treatment protocol according to Massicotte et al. [27]. In this study the beneficial effect of LMWH was demonstrated in acute thrombotic occlusions of different locations. Furthermore, the pharmocodynamics of anti-Xa activity at the LMWH dosages administered was assessed in our patient group to investigate whether effective levels can be reached over a sufficient period of time and whether the LMWH enoxaparin can be given for prophylaxis over a prolonged period without causing adverse effects.

Patients and Methods

In the 8-year period from 1996 to 2004, we conducted a prospective follow-up study on children with DVT including SVT admitted to the University Children's Hospital of the Martin Luther University Halle-Wittenberg for treatment of thrombosis.

All patients were exclusively treated with enoxaparin (Clexane®), with an initial dosage of 1.0 mg/kg of body weight, administered twice daily. For neonates an increased dosage of 1.5 mg/kg of body weight twice daily was used [27]. Anti-Xa activity in the plasma was first measured 4 h after the third application of enoxaparin. Further measurements were taken every 2 days within the first 14 days, thereafter 1–2 times per week until the end of the 4th week of treatment. Dosage adaptations were performed immediately to reach a stable, therapeutically relevant anti-Xa activity within a range of 0.5–0.8 U/ml. Anti-Xa activity was determined by a chromogen method provided by Dade Behring, Marburg, Germany. In the first 4 weeks we carried out an average of 10 determinations per patient (range 7–12). D-dimers were measured in parallel by turbidometry (Dade Behring).

To verify the response to the therapy, i.e. ascertaining the recanalization of the affected vessels upon therapy, imaging methods such as duplex sonography, MRI or CT [36, 53, 57] have been performed in addition to clinical examination.

In patients with SVT, MR angiography was performed initially and at 3, 6 and 12 months of follow-up and in yearly intervals thereafter. In patients with DVT duplex sonography was used more frequently. During the first 4 weeks of therapy checks were conducted once a week, later on every 4 weeks over a period of 6 months after the start of treatment. Thereafter, checks were performed every 6 months.

Monitoring of anti-Xa activity has been performed to assess the optimal dosage of enoxaparin for treatment of thrombosis in our patient group. This was only studied in patients who had been treated and documented according to protocol.

Asymptomatic and symptomatic venous rethrombosis, affirmed by an objective examination method, as well as hemorrhages, heparin-induced thrombocytopenia (HIT), compliance problems and death were all end points of this follow-up.

Results

A total of 40 pediatric patients suffering from differently located venous thromboses were treated in a single pediatric thrombosis unit. Twenty-seven of 40 patients were treated according to protocol and were prospectively followed up. Seventeen patients suffered from DVT and 10 from SVT, regardless of whether there was only one affected vessel or whether there were several affected vessels in anatomically neighboring regions.

In contrast to adults, DVT affected the lower half of the body in 47% of cases (table 1). The mean age of the DVT patients was 10.3 years (range 0.1–16) and 10.9 years in SVT patients (range 0.1–16). In contrast to the SVT patients, where there was no particular prevalence

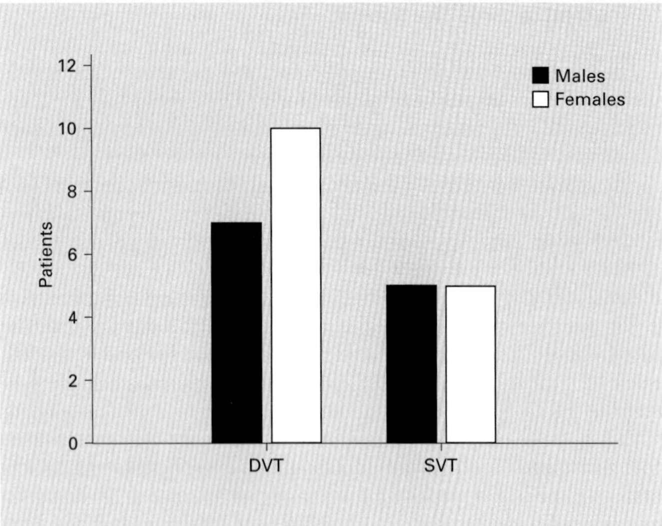

Fig. 1. No particular prevalence of gender in SVT patients and predominance of females in DVT patients.

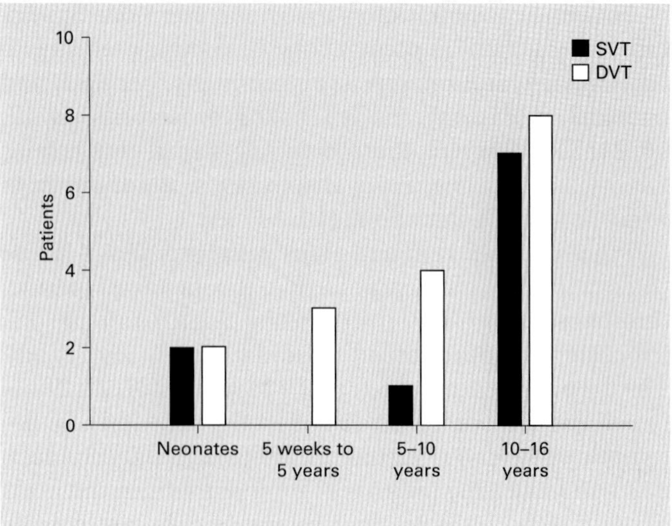

Fig. 2. Distribution of age in DVT and SVT patients.

Table 1. Localization of DVT (n = 17)

	n
Iliacal-femoropopliteal axis	8
Vena jugularis interna	3
Vena brachiocephalica	2
Vena subclavia	2
Vena cava inferior	2

Table 2. Cause of thrombosis

	%
Malignancy	40
Spontaneous	26
Postoperative	11
Posttraumatic	4
Postinflammatory	8
Other	11

of gender; a predominance of females was found in cases of DVT (fig. 1). Considering our selective group of patients in a university children's hospital, most events involving SVT and DVT were found in patients between 10 and 16 years of age (fig. 2).

In 40% of cases thrombotic events occurred within the scope of a malignant disease, which therefore represented the largest group. Besides them, there were 25% of spontaneous thrombotic occlusions without causative accompanying diseases. In the remainder there were postoperative, posttraumatic and postinflammatory occlusions (table 2). Further details on the cause of the DVT and SVT are given in figures 3 and 4. SVT occurred more frequently during the induction phase of the chemotherapy for acute lymphatic leukemia and non-Hodgkin lymphoma. Both of these malignant diseases were treated according to BFM protocols (ALL-BFM 1995/ALL-BFM 2000/ NHL-BFM 1995). A total of 5 cases were observed. Further analysis showed that the application of the protein inhibitor *L*-asparaginase was followed by a massive fall of the anticoagulatory protein antithrombin III as well as of fibrinogen in these 5 patients. In 10 cases (37%) we were able to ascertain one or several additional genetic prothrombotic risk factors, such as FV G1691A mutation, prothrombin G20210A mutation or a homozygous 4G/4G genotype in the plasminogen activator inhibitor-1 (fig. 5). In further cases (n = 6) we were also able to determine additional exogenous factors such as nicotine abuse or the use of oral contraception (fig. 6).

If necessary, the dosage was adapted immediately, most of all during the 1st week of treatment. The final mean dosage during the therapeutic phase of enoxaparin treatment was 1.175 mg/kg of body weight (range 1.05–1.38), administered twice daily, thus achieving a mean anti-Xa activity of 0.61 U/ml (range 0.51–0.78) (fig. 7). Therapeutically effective levels were reached from the

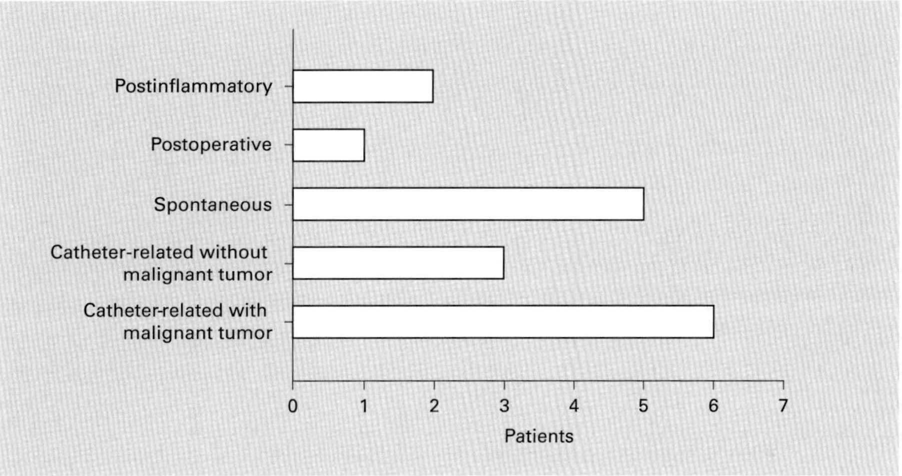

Fig. 3. Presumable causes of DVT.

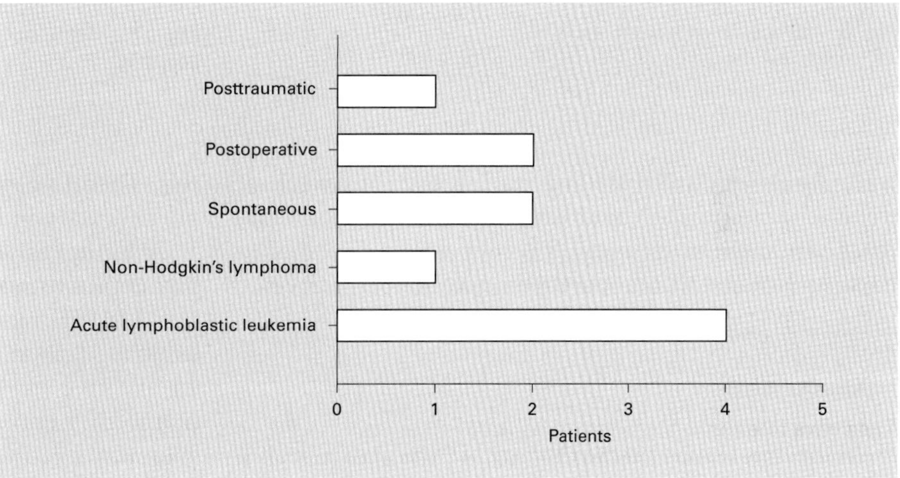

Fig. 4. Presumable causes of SVT.

2nd day of treatment onwards. Upon this therapy, 85.2% of the patients responded well to enoxaparin therapy achieving a reopening of their vessels. The mean duration of the therapeutic phase was 16.5 days (range 10–24), which was followed by prophylaxis using enoxaparin at a dosage of 1 mg/kg of body weight daily for a mean of 9.8 months (range 5–24). In addition, 23 of 27 patients showed complete (n = 15; 55.6%) or partial (n = 8; 29.6%) patency of the affected vessels. During therapy, D-dimers did not reincrease in any case. No rethrombosis was observed during a follow-up period of a mean of 2.3 years (range 0.5–6.25).

The course of 4 newborns was analyzed separately. Patients of this cohort received a higher LMWH dosage (1.54 mg/kg of body weight 2 × per day) in order to obtain the target anti-Xa activity (0.64 U/ml) (fig. 7).

In this pilot study no thrombotic event required primary surgical intervention. One patient experienced in-

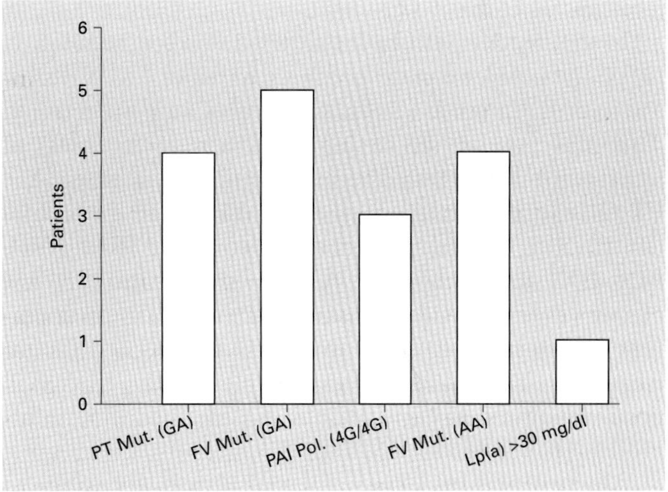

Fig. 5. Genetic prothrombotic risk factors (one or several additional). PT = Prothrombin; Mut. = mutation; PAI = plasminogen activator inhibitor; Pol = polymorphism; Lp(a) = lipoprotein (a).

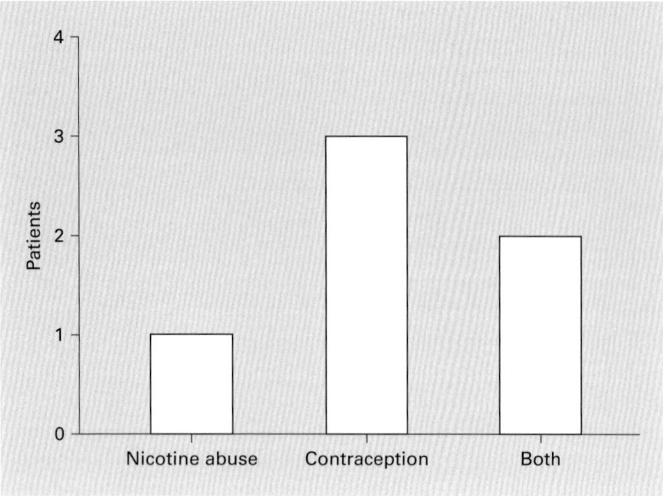

Fig. 6. Additional exogenous factors.

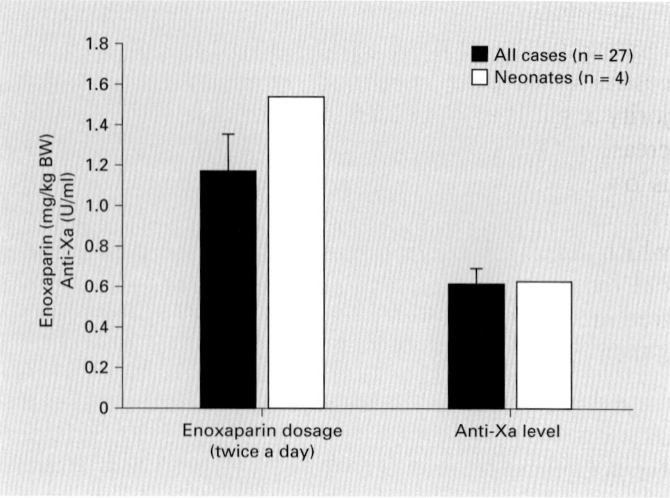

Fig. 7. Mean enoxaparin dosage and mean anti-Xa activity achieved.

tracerebral subdural bleeding during the 2nd week of treatment requiring neurosurgical intervention and reached complete recovery. Further adverse events or heparin-induced thrombocytopenia were not observed.

Discussion

In this pilot study on the therapy of thrombosis in children patency of the affected vessel could be achieved in a high number of patients treated with LMWH using a sufficiently high dosage reaching anti-Xa activity between 0.6 and 0.7 U/ml.

In agreement with case studies described previously [27, 34, 44, 48], neonates required a higher LMWH dosage in order to reach a sufficient level of anti-Xa activity. This may possibly be explained by a relative excess of antithrombin compared to prothrombin (increased AT: PT ratio) upon treatment with LMWH, since the factors contributing to the prothrombin complex (FII, FVII, FIX, FX) are physiologically lower during the first few months of life. In addition, a different distribution pattern in reference to body weight as well as a different clearance of LMWH are responsible for the increased dosage required in early infancy as described in animals models [6, 15, 38–43, 45–47].

Albeit a higher dosage of LMWH was necessary to achieve a comparable anti-Xa activity in newborns it is unknown whether this activity is required to reach therapeutic success, i.e. the patency rates of the affected vessels. Therefore, it cannot be concluded that higher doses are necessary in neonates.

A further advantage of LMWH application lies in the higher profibrinolytic effect. Previous studies have shown that LMWH has a high potential to release endothelial-associated tissue factor pathway inhibitor [59] leading to an additive on the thrombus. This effect is most pronounced in enoxaparin. Furthermore, the target level is achieved rapidly which can be explained by the high bioavailability of enoxaparin [58, 59]. Throughout the period of treatment, levels of anti-Xa activity remained at the target level in 95% of the children.

Hematologic malignancy was the most frequent underlying disease in our patient group. Especially upon *L*-asparaginase therapy venous thrombosis occurred in patients with acute lymphatic leukemia (protocol I: ALL-BFM) and with B-non-Hodgkin lymphoma (protocol I: – NHL-BFM). A high prothrombotic risk induced by asparaginase therapy has been described by several authors [9, 17–20, 22–25].

The recommendations given for the treatment of adults were transferable to pediatric patients in terms of dosage and anti-Xa activity achieved. Treatment was safe in neonates as well. During treatment with therapeutic dosages, measurement of anti-Xa activity is of major importance. Our experience clearly demonstrates that adaptation of the dosage was necessary to avoid too high levels of anti-Xa activity, which possibly results in a higher bleeding risk. A cumulative effect of enoxaparin has hitherto not been described although it certainly needs to be discussed.

In conclusion, administration of enoxaparin produced therapeutically effective anti-Xa activities leading to successful recanalization of thrombotic vessels in the vast majority of patients. Reocclusion of the blood vessels or reincrease of D-dimers was not observed. The risk of bleeding is low if the dosage is adapted measuring the anti-Xa activity. The treatment requires only minimal monitoring, which makes it possible to treat neonates and infants without frequent venous punctures; they are required in the treatment with unfractioned heparins in order to achieve a therapeutically effective PTT adjustment.

Acknowledgement

We thank U. Nowak-Göttl and Sabine Thedieck from the Department of Paediatric Haematology/Oncology, University Children's Hospital Münster, for providing laboratory data about genetic prothrombotic markers as well as for helpful discussions in the preparation of the manuscript. In addition, we thank Aventis Pharma Germany for supporting this study.

References

1 Andrew M: Developmental hemostasis: relevance to thromboembolic complications in pediatric patients. Thromb Haemost 1995;74: 415–425.

2 Gurgey A, Balta G, Gumruk F, Altay C: Analysis of some clinical and laboratory aspects of adolescent patients with thrombosis. Blood Coagul Fibrinolysis 2004;15:657–662.

3 Casais P, Meschengieser SS, Gennari LC, Alberto MF, Sanchez-Luceros A, Blanco AN, Lazzari MA: Morbidity of lupus anticoagulants in children: a single institution experience. Thromb Res 2004;114:245–249.

4 Obermoser G, Bitterlich W, Kunz F, Sepp NT: Clinical significance of anticardiolipin and anti-beta2-glycoprotein I antibodies. Int Arch Allergy Immunol 2004;135:148–153.

5 Massicotte MP, Dix D, Monagle P, Adams M, Andrew M: Central venous catheter related thrombosis in children: analysis of the Canadian Registry of Venous Thromboembolic Complications. J Pediatr 1998;133:770–776.

6 Schmidt B, Andrew M: Neonatal thrombosis: report of a prospective Canadian and international registry. Pediatrics 1995;96:939–943.

7 Glaser DW, Medeiros D, Rollins N, Buchanan GR: Catheter-related thrombosis in children with cancer. J Pediatr 2001;138:255–259.

8 Molinari AC, Castagnola E, Mazzola C, Piacentino M, Fratino G: Thromboembolic complications related to indwelling central venous catheters in children with oncological/haematological diseases: a retrospective study of 362 catheters. Support Care Cancer 2001;9:539–544.

9 Mitchell L, Hoogendoorn H, Giles AR, Vegh P, Andrew M: Increased endogenous thrombin generation in children with acute lymphoblastic leukemia: risk of thrombotic complications in L'Asparaginase-induced antithrombin III deficiency. Blood 1994;83:386–391.

10 Lane DA, Grant PJ: Role of hemostatic gene polymorphisms in venous and arterial thrombotic disease. Blood 2000;95:1517–1532.

11 Junker R, Koch HG, Auberger K, Munchow N, Ehrenforth S, Nowak-Gottl U: Prothrombin G20210A gene mutation and further prothrombotic risk factors in childhood thrombophilia. Arterioscler Thromb Vasc Biol 1999;19: 2568–2572.

12 Nowak-Gottl U, Junker R, Hartmeier M, Koch HG, Munchow N, Assmann G, von Eckardstein A: Increased lipoprotein(a) is an important risk factor for venous thromboembolism in childhood. Circulation 1999;100:743–748.

13 Vielhaber H, Ehrenforth S, Koch HG, Scharrer I, van der Werf N, Nowak-Gottl U: Cerebral venous sinus thrombosis in infancy and childhood: role of genetic and acquired risk factors of thrombophilia. Eur J Pediatr 1998;157: 555–560.

14 deVeber G, Andrew M; Canadian Pediatric Ischemic Stroke Study Group: Cerebral sinovenous thrombosis in children. N Engl J Med 2001;345:417–423.

15 Andrew M, Vegh P, Johnston M, Bowker J, Ofosu F, Mitchell L: Maturation of the hemostatic system during childhood. Blood 1992; 80:1998–2005.

16 Ruud E, Holmstrom H, Natvig S, Wesenberg F: Prevalence of thrombophilia and central venous catheter-associated neck vein thrombosis in 41 children with cancer – a prospective study. Med Pediatr Oncol 2002;38:405–410.

17 Homans AC, Rybak ME, Baglini RL, Tiarks C, Steiner ME, Forman EN: Effect of *L*-asparaginase administration on coagulation and platelet function in children with leukaemia. J Clin Oncol 1987;5:811–817.

18 Semeraro N, Montemurro P, Giordano P, Schettini F, Santoro N, De Mattia D, Giordano D, Conese M, Colucci M: Unbalanced coagulation-fibrinolysis potential during *L*-asparaginase therapy in children with acute lymphoblastic leukaemia. Thromb Haemost 1990;64: 38–40.

19 Miniero R, Saracco P, Einaudi S, Garofalo F, Lange MM, Madon E: *L*-Asparaginase-induced coagulopathy in children with acute lymphoblastic leukaemia. Drugs Exp Clin Res 1987;13:377–379.

20 Shapiro AD, Clarke SL, Christian JM, Odom LF, Hathaway WE: Thrombosis in children receiving *L*-asparaginase. Determining patients at risk. Am J Pediatr Hematol Oncol 1993;15: 400–405.

21 Reddingius RE, Patte C, Couanet D, Kalifa C, Lemerle J: Dural sinus thrombosis in children with cancer. Med Pediatr Oncol 1997;29:296–302.

22 Heller C, Heinecke A, Junker R, Knofler R, Kosch A, Kurnik K, Schobess R, von Eckardstein A, Strater R, Zieger B, Nowak-Gottl U; Childhood Stroke Study Group: Cerebral venous thrombosis in children: a multifactorial origin. Circulation 2003;108:1362–1367.

23 Mauz-Korholz C, Junker R, Gobel U, Nowak-Gottl U: Prothrombotic risk factors in children with acute lymphoblastic leukemia treated with delayed *E. coli* asparaginase (COALL-92 and 97 protocols). Thromb Haemost 2000;83: 840–843.

24 Nowak-Gottl U, Heinecke A, von Kries R, Nurnberger W, Munchow N, Junker R: Thrombotic events revisited in children with acute lymphoblastic leukemia: impact of concomitant *Escherichia coli* asparaginase/prednisone administration. Thromb Res 2001;103:165–172.

25 Nowak-Gottl U, Ahlke E, Fleischhack G, Schwabe D, Schobess R, Schumann C, Junker R: Thromboembolic events in children with acute lymphoblastic leukemia (BFM protocols): prednisone versus dexamethasone administration. Blood 2003;101:2529–2533.

26 Massicotte P, Julian JA, Gent M, Shields K, Marzinotto V, Szechtman B, Andrew M; REVIVE Study Group: An open-label randomized controlled trial of low molecular weight heparin compared to heparin and coumadin for the treatment of venous thromboembolic events in children: the REVIVE trial. Thromb Res 2003;109:85–92.

27 Massicotte P, Adams M, Marzinotto V, Brooker LA, Andrew M: Low-molecular-weight heparin in pediatric patients with thrombotic disease: a dose finding study. J Pediatr 1996;128: 313–318.

28 Sutor AH, Massicotte P, Leaker M, Andrew M: Heparin therapy in pediatric patients. Semin Thromb Hemost 1997;23:303–319.

29 deVeber G, Chan A, Monagle P, Marzinotto V, Armstrong D, Massicotte P, Leaker M, Andrew M: Anticoagulation therapy in pediatric patients with sinovenous thrombosis: a cohort study. Arch Neurol 1998;55:1533–1537.

30 Massicotte MP: Low-molecular-weight heparin therapy in children. J Pediatr Hematol Oncol 2000;22:98–99.

31 Dix D, Andrew M, Marzinotto V, Charpentier K, Bridge S, Monagle P, deVeber G, Leaker M, Chan AK, Massicotte MP: The use of low molecular weight heparin in pediatric patients: a prospective cohort study. J Pediatr 2000;136: 439–445.

32 Massicotte P, Julian JA, Gent M, Shields K, Marzinotto V, Szechtman B, Andrew M; REVIVE Study Group: An open-label randomized controlled trial of low molecular weight heparin compared to heparin and coumadin for the treatment of venous thromboembolic events in children: the REVIVE trial. Thromb Res 2003;109:85–92.

33 Massicotte P, Julian JA, Marzinotto V, Gent M, Shields K, Chan AK, Szechtman B, Kohne S, Shepherd S, Bacher P, Andrew M: Dose-finding and pharmacokinetic profiles of prophylactic doses of a low molecular weight heparin (reviparin-sodium) in pediatric patients. Thromb Res 2003;109:93–99.

34 Streif W, Goebel G, Chan AK, Massicotte MP: Use of low molecular mass heparin (enoxaparin) in newborn infants: a prospective cohort study of 62 patients. Arch Dis Child Fetal Neonatal Ed 2003;88:F365–F370.

35 Levy DM, Massicotte MP, Harvey E, Hebert D, Silverman ED: Thromboembolism in paediatric lupus patients. Lupus 2003;12:741–746.

36 Revel-Vilk S, Sharathkumar A, Massicotte P, Marzinotto V, Daneman A, Dix D, Chan A: Natural history of arterial and venous thrombosis in children treated with low molecular weight heparin: a longitudinal study by ultrasound. J Thromb Haemost 2004;2:42–46.

37 Sutor AH, Chan AK, Massicotte P: Low-molecular-weight heparin in pediatric patients. Semin Thromb Hemost 2004;30(suppl 1):31–39.

38 Anton N, Massicotte MP: Venous thromboembolism in pediatrics. Semin Vasc Med 2001;1: 111–122.

39 Andrew M: Developmental hemostasis: relevance to hemostatic problems during childhood. Semin Thromb Hemost 1995;21:341–356.

40 Beardsley DS: Hemostasis in the perinatal period: approach to the diagnosis of coagulation disorders. Semin Perinatol 1991;15(3 suppl 2):25–34.

41 Nowak-Gottl U, Kosch A, Schlegel N: Neonatal thromboembolism. Semin Thromb Hemost 2003;29:227–234.

42 Nowak-Gottl U, Kosch A, Schlegel N, Salem M, Manco-Johnson M: Thromboembolism in children. Curr Opin Hematol 2002;9:448–453.

43 Nowak-Gottl U, Kosch A, Schlegel N: Thromboembolism in newborns, infants and children. Thromb Haemost 2001;86:464–474.

44 Ho SH, Wu JK, Hamilton DP, Dix DB, Wadsworth LD: An assessment of published pediatric dosage guidelines for enoxaparin: a retrospective review. J Pediatr Hematol Oncol 2004;26:561–566.

45 Michaels LA, Gurian M, Hegyi T, Drachtman RA : Low molecular weight heparin in the treatment of venous and arterial thromboses in the premature infant. Pediatrics 2004;114: 703–707.

46 Vieira A, Berry L, Ofosu F, Andrew M: Heparin sensitivity and resistance in the neonate: an explanation. Thromb Res 1991;63:85–98.

47 Andrew M, Ofosu F, Brooker L, Buchanan MR: The comparison of the pharmacokinetics of a low molecular weight heparin in the newborn and adult pig. Thromb Res 1989;56:529–539.

48 Albisetti M, Andrew M: Low molecular weight heparin in children. Eur J Pediatr 2002;161: 71–77.

49 Hofmann S, Knoefler R, Lorenz N, Siegert G, Wendisch J, Mueller D, Taut-Sack H, Dinger J, Kabus M: Clinical experiences with low-molecular weight heparins in pediatric patients. Thromb Res 2001;103:345–353.

50 Manco-Johnson MJ, Nuss R, Hays T, Krupski W, Drose J, Manco-Johnson ML: Combined thrombolytic and anticoagulant therapy for venous thrombosis in children. J Pediatr 2000; 136:446–453.

51 Kosch A, Kuwertz-Broking E, Heller C, Kurnik K, Schobess R, Nowak-Gottl U: Renal venous thrombosis in neonates: prothrombotic risk factors and long-term follow-up. Blood 2004; 104:1356–1360.

52 Shevell MI, Silver K, O'Gorman AM, Watters GV, Montes JL: Neonatal dural sinus thrombosis. Pediatr Neurol 1989;5:161–165.

53 West WM, Brady-West D: Ultrasonography of the lower limbs for deep vein thrombosis at the University Hospital of the West Indies. A five-year analysis. West Indian Med J 2002;51:35–36.

54 Giannoukas AD, Fatouros M, Batsis H, Mitsis M, Matsagas M, Koulouras V, Tsampoulas C, Kappas M, Cassioumis A: Symptomatic deep venous thrombosis of the lower limb. Int Angiol 1998;17:151–154.

55 Andrew M, David M, Adams M, Ali K, Anderson R, Barnard D, Bernstein M, Brisson L, Cairney B, DeSai D, et al: Venous thromboembolic complications (VTE) in children: first analyses of the Canadian Registry of VTE. Blood 1994;83:1251–1257.

56 Manco-Johnson MJ, Grabowski EF, Hellgreen M, Kemahli AS, Massicotte MP, Muntean W, Peters M, Schlegel N, Wang M, Nowak-Gottl U: Recommendations for tPA thrombolysis in children. On behalf of the Scientific Subcommittee on Perinatal and Pediatric Thrombosis of the Scientific and Standardization Committee of the International Society of Thrombosis and Haemostasis. Thromb Haemost 2002;88: 157–158.

57 Connor SE, Jarosz JM: Magnetic resonance imaging of cerebral venous sinus thrombosis. Clin Radiol 2002;57:449–461.

58 Ip BK, Thomson AR, Moriarty HAT: A comparison of the sensitivity of APTT reagents to the effects of enoxaparin, a low-molecular weight heparin. Pathology 2001;33:347–352.

59 Koppenhagen K: Enoxaparin – Im Zeichen der Unverwechselbarkeit. Klinikarzt 2004;33(suppl):8–9.

Acta Haematologica

Acta Haematol 2006;115:237–247
DOI: 10.1159/000090941

Safety and Efficacy of Danaparoid (Orgaran®) Use in Children

Christoph Bidlingmaier[a] Harry N. Magnani[c] Monika Girisch[b] Karin Kurnik[a]

[a]Department of Paediatric Haemostaseology, Dr. von Hauner's University Children's Hospital, Munich, and
[b]Department of Cardiology, University Hospital for Children and Adolescents, Tübingen, Germany;
[c]Clinical Consultant to Organon International BV, Oss, The Netherlands

Key Words
Danaparoid · Heparin-induced thrombocytopenia, therapy

Abstract
Immune-mediated heparin-induced thrombocytopenia (HIT) is an uncommon but serious complication of therapy with heparins. It affects all ages and requires replacement of the causative anticoagulant. However, information on alternative antithrombotic use in children with HIT is limited. This paper reviews 27 published and 7 unpublished case reports of children aged 2 weeks to 17 years treated with danaparoid. Thirty-three suffered from HIT or suspected HIT, and 1 child without HIT had a high bleeding risk. All children had severe underlying problems increasing their thrombotic and/or bleeding risk. HIT diagnosis was confirmed serologically or clinically in 26 cases (78.8%). Danaparoid regimens were similar to those used in adults, but in general, younger children needed higher daily doses of danaparoid to achieve the same target plasma anti-Xa levels than teenagers or adults. Of those with a known outcome 28/33 children (84.8%) survived, 7 having suffered from a serious adverse event. Five deaths occurred including 1 thrombotic and 2 major bleeds. Three of the in total 4 major bleeding events occurred in children undergoing surgery with cardiopulmonary bypass. We conclude that despite the reported adverse events danaparoid can be used as an alternative antithrombotic for children who are intolerant of the heparins, except in cases requiring cardiopulmonary bypass surgery.

Introduction

The antithrombotic agent danaparoid (Orgaran®) is a heparinoid (molecular weight on average 6,000 Da). Its antithrombotic activity is mediated predominantly by anti-Xa activity, which has a plasma half-life of approximately 24 h in adults, but its antithrombotic activity has a half-life of about 7 h. Danaparoid does not possess thrombolytic properties and there is no antidote. Clinical trials began in 1981 and at the same time it was also made available for the treatment of patients with intolerance to unfractionated and/or low-molecular-weight (LMW) heparin, particularly heparin-induced thrombocytopenia (HIT), in a compassionate-use program (CUP) for named patients [1, 2]. It was first approved for the use in adult patients with a risk of deep vein thrombosis (DVT) in 1991 and since in vitro cross-reactivity with the heparin-induced antiplatelet antibody was reported to be low (6.3%) [2], for those suffering from HIT in 1994. Currently danaparoid is available in Europe, Canada, Australia and New Zealand, but not in the US, for the indication HIT and in Japan for treatment of disseminated intravascular coagulation (DIC). Although efficacy and

KARGER

Fax +41 61 306 12 34
E-Mail karger@karger.ch
www.karger.com

0001–5792/06/1154–0237$23.50/0

Accessible online at:
www.karger.com/aha

Dr. Christoph Bidlingmaier
Dr. von Hauner's University Children's Hospital, Dept. of Paediatric Haemostaseology
Lindwurmstrasse 4, DE–80337 Munich (Germany)
Tel. +49 89 5160 2811, Fax +49 89 5160 4453
E-Mail christoph.bidlingmaier@med.uni-muenchen.de

safety of danaparoid have not been established in children it is the most frequently reported drug used for the treatment of pediatric HIT [3]. HIT is an uncommon, immune-mediated, potentially serious complication of (LMW) heparin therapy [4]. The reported incidence of HIT in adults approaches 5% [5]; it appears to be less frequent in children [6, 7]. HIT and other forms of (LMW) heparin intolerance require the use of alternative antithrombotic agents. The purpose of this review is to analyze the use of danaparoid in children with HIT and other reasons for alternative anticoagulation and draw conclusions concerning its suitability.

Methods

MEDLINE and conference proceedings were searched for details of danaparoid use in children (age 0–17 years inclusive) from 1981 to May 2004. Cases reported directly to the manufacturer were added to these, either as part of the CUP or as spontaneous adverse event reports, and previously unpublished cases of the authors.

Event Confirmation

DVT was usually confirmed by compression ultrasound and pulmonary emboli by ventilation/perfusion quotient (V/Q) or computerized tomography (CT) scans. Peripheral arterial thromboses were identified mainly by clinical evidence of ischemia and CT scans were used for intracardiac thromboses. In some cases, no data were available.

HIT Diagnosis

HIT was suspected if an unexpected platelet count reduction of 30% or more and/or thrombosis occurred usually >5 days after starting the patient on heparin therapy. Confirmation was usually sought by one of the following serological methods: platelet aggregation test (PAT) [8], heparin-induced platelet activation (HIPAA) assay [9], enzyme-linked immunosorbent assay (EIA) [10], serotonin release assay [11] and immune fluorescence assay [12]. In some patients the serological test(s) used was negative, but the diagnosis was further strengthened by observing that the platelet count dropped by 50% or more with no other obvious cause, or rechallenge thrombocytopenia occurred, e.g. each time heparin was administered for hemodialysis. In some cases, no serological data were available. The same serological methods used for HIT diagnosis in each patient were also used for testing for danaparoid cross-reactivity.

Danaparoid Dosing and Monitoring

The danaparoid administration schedules recommended for similar presenting clinical situations in adults [2] were used. Nevertheless, the danaparoid dosing intensity for particular clinical situations was determined for each child by target plasma anti-Xa activity intervals monitored using the amidolytic plasma anti-factor-Xa activity assay of Teien and Lie [13], modified for use with danaparoid. Anti-Xa activity intervals were based on those used for adults: 0.15–0.4 U/ml for routine thrombosis prophylaxis and 0.4–0.8 U/ml for thrombosis treatment and during hemodialysis.

Criteria for Judging the Outcome of Danaparoid Treatment

An adequate clinical outcome of danaparoid treatment included all of the following:

1 Platelet count recovery defined as counts increasing to above $100 \times 10^9/l$ for patients transferred early (within a few days despite no adverse event occurring) to a vitamin K antagonist (VKA) or to above $150 \times 10^9/l$ for those remaining on danaparoid.
2 Lack of a clinically significant change in a normal platelet count in nonthrombocytopenic patients with confirmed or suspected HIT.
3 Absence of new, progressive or recurrent thrombosis (unless a new thrombosis was treated by increasing the daily dose of danaparoid).
4 Stabilization or improvement of ischemia.
5 Survival without or despite minor adverse events such as minor bleeding, e.g. from venipuncture site or postoperatively, particularly if danaparoid therapy was continued.
6 Amputation for clinical ischemia already present at danaparoid treatment initiation, which is reported not to have progressed further.

Non-thrombotic- or non-bleeding-associated deaths clearly due to the underlying disease are not considered due to danaparoid if the above criteria were also satisfied in the reports.

An inadequate clinical outcome of danaparoid treatment included any of the following:

1 Need to discontinue danaparoid prematurely because of a nonfatal event (usually major bleeding, suspected or confirmed danaparoid cross-reactivity or other serious adverse event reportedly attributed to danaparoid).
2 Death due to thrombotic or bleeding complications or for 'unknown/unspecified' reason.

Results

Patient Population

Thirty-four detailed unique case reports of danaparoid use in children have been traced: 4 unpublished cases from the CUP (cases 19, 20, 21 and 22), 1 patient from the same program (case 26), but published separately [14], 3 previously unpublished cases of the authors (cases 3, 23 and 24), 1 in an MD thesis (case 17) [15] and 25 from 15 independent publications [12, 16–29]. Detailed data on these patients, presenting features, treatment and outcome are shown in table 1 and summarized in table 2. Case 6 [18] was treated on two separate occasions.

Reasons for Danaparoid Use

Danaparoid was used to treat 24 children with confirmed HIT, 9 with suspected HIT and 1 non-HIT patient with a high bleeding risk who required hemodialysis. The primary reasons for danaparoid use in these children (see table 1) were routine thromboprophylaxis in 6 cases, thrombosis treatment in 9 cases (some of whom contin-

Table 1. Summary of patients treated with danaparoid: presenting features, treatment and outcome

No.	Gender, age, BW	Diagnosis at hospital admission	Thrombophilia	Complications of HIT	HIT diagnosis	Danaparoid dosage	Treatment duration, days	Outcome[a]	Action	Authors
1	M, 14 mo, 9.2 kg	Fallot's teralogy, VACTERL		TP after previous surgery	serology +	for cardiac catheterization: 30 U/kg bolus i.v. + 2–5 U/kg/h i.v.	2	recovered		Girisch et al. [12]
2	M, 11 y	cerebrovascular malformation	APL	TP	serology +	for prophylaxis: 20 U/kg bolus i.v. + 10 U/kg/d s.c.	4	recovered		Bocquet et al. [16]
3	M, 1 mo, 3.5 kg	hypoplastic left heart		TP	serology +	for prophylaxis: 8–70 U/kg/d	16	recovered		unpubl. case, Girisch
4	M, 15 y, 118 kg	appendectomy, DVT right leg	PSD	iliac vein thrombosis	serology +, cross-reactivity –	for treatment: 17 U/kg bolus i.v. + 3.7–1.7 U/kg/h rt-PA	10	minor bleed	stop rt-PA, recovered (recanalization)	Klement et al. [17]
5	M 10 y, 25 kg	end-stage renal failure, hemodialysis		ECC clots, RDS, TP	rechallenge +, serology –	mean predialysis: 84 U/kg bolus i.v.	548	recovered		Neuhaus et al. [18]
6	M, 14 y, 35 kg	end-stage renal failure, hemodialysis		ECC clots, chest pain, TP	rechallenge +, serology –	mean predialysis: 85 U/kg bolus i.v.	183	recovered		Neuhaus et al. [18]
7	M, 12 y, 60 kg	DVT left leg	ANA +	arterial TE	serology possibly + cross-reactivity +	for treatment: 5–8.3 U/kg/h	1	(TP recovered)	switch to lepirudin, forefoot amputation, recovered	Schiffmann et al. [19]
8	M, 17 y	rhabdomyosarcoma, chemotherapy		TP, cutaneous and nose bleeds	serology +	for prophylaxis: 20 U/kg/d for line flush: 750 U in 5 ml saline	1	recovered		Sauer et al. [20]
9	M, 14 y	mitral valve tumors, femoral artery emboli		amaurosis fugax, TP	serology +	before surgery: 5,000 U bolus i.v. (BW unknown) postsurgery: 0.6–1.2 U/kg/h i.v.	9	recovered		Wilhelm et al. [22]
10	F, 2 y, 12 kg	single ventricle, Fontan surgery	APL	DVT, conduit thrombosis	serology +, cross-reactivity –	before second Fontan surgery: 30 U/kg bolus i.v. + 2 U/kg/h during surgery: 62 U/kg bolus i.v. + 4 U/ml into prime + 125 U/kg bolus i.v. postsurgery: 4–6 U/kg/h	>3	major bleed, transient increase AST and serum lactate	reoperation recovered (recanalization)	Saxon et al. [28]
11	F, 17 y	right atrial thrombus, DVT + PE	APL	TP	unknown	for treatment: 80–150 U/h (BW unknown)	n/a	recovered		Weigel et al. [21]
12	F, 7 mo, 5 kg	CHD, renal insufficiency, SDH		thrombus on pulmonary valve	unknown	for peritoneal dialysis: 0.2–0.5 U/kg/h i.v.	8	suspected pulmonary bleed, died		Weigel et al. [21]
13	F, 13 y	DVT + PE, cardiac shock, thrombus right ventricle	APL PCD	recurrent PE, intracardiac thrombi, DVT	serology +, cross-reactivity –	for treatment: 1.2–3.4 U/kg/h	25	ICT regression, late DVT	switch to lepirudin, recovered	Zöhrer et al. [23]
14	M, 12 y	DVT left leg	APL PSD	DVT, TP, IVC thrombosis,	serology +, cross-reactivity –	for treatment: 20.8 U/kg bolus i.v. + 6.7–2.7 U/kg/h i.v.	16	recovered (partial recanalization)		Zöhrer et al. [23]
15	M 10 y	arterial thrombosis left leg	APL PSD ANA HLP IIa	arterial TE (left toes), TP	serology +, cross-reactivity –	for treatment: 5.4 U/kg/h for 22 d and 2.7 U/kg/h for 8 d	30	ischemia stabilized	on VKA, amputation of toes, recovered	Zöhrer et al. [23]
16	M, 9 y	DVT femoral veins	APL PSD	TP	serology +, cross-reactivity –	for treatment: 28.6 U/kg bolus i.v. + 7.1–2.9 U/kg/h i.v.	9	recovery (partial recanalization)		Zöhrer et al. [23]
17	M, 16 y, 90 kg	accident victim	APL	TP	serology +, cross-reactivity –	for prophylaxis: 8.3 U/kg/d s.c.	7	recovered		Barth [15]
18	M, 7 mo	premature birth, RDS, DIC	ATD	TP	serology +	for prophylaxis: 2.0–4.0 U/kg/h i.v.	9	new TP	switch to lepirudin (TP persisted)	Nguyen et al. [24]
19	M, 16 y, 40 kg	reflux nephropathy, renal failure, dialysis, cardiomyopathy		ECC clots	serology +, cross-reactivity +	prehemodialysis: 112–175 U/kg bolus i.v. predialysis	1	circuit clotting	dialysis abandoned	unpublished case 223, CUP

Table 1 (continued)

No.	Gender, age, BW	Diagnosis at hospital admission	Thrombo-philia	Complications of HIT	HIT diagnosis	Danaparoid dosage	Treatment duration, days	Outcome[a]	Action	Authors
20	F, 16 y	cardiomyopathy, heart transplantation		PE	unknown	for prophylaxis: 1,250 U bolus + 312–150 U/h i.v. for cardiac transplant: 7,500 U postthoracotomy 5,000 U into prime and 1,500 U intraoperatively	5 1	major	multiple transfusions, recovered	unpubl. case 357, CUP
21	F, 7 y, 27 kg	Fallot's tetralogy, hepatic vein thrombosis		TP	serology + cross-reactivity –	for prophylaxis: unknown for line flush: 70 U/l saline	19 18	sepsis, MOF, new TP (inadvertent UFH administration), died	seroconversion, test negative	unpubl. case 418, CUP
22	M, 1 y, 6.5 kg	Fallot's tetralogy, septicemia, renal failure, dialysis		TP	serology +	for peritoneal dialysis: 0.5 U/kg/h into diaysate + 1.8 U/kg/h i.v.	>14	recovered		unpubl. case 625, CUP
23	M, 13 y, 40 kg	multiple DVT + PE (no benefit from lysis or other LMWH)		TP	serology –, clinical +	for treatment: up to 19 U/kg s.c. twice daily, used in part with rt-PA	57	recovery (partial recanalization)		unpubl. case Bidlingmaier, Kurnik
24	F, 2 mo, 3.3 kg	CHD for surgery		TP	serology –, clinical +	for treatment and during surgery: up to 8.0 U/kg/h	37	major bleed during surgery, died		unpubl. case Girisch
25	M, 10 mo 4.33 kg	premature birth, VACTERL sequence		TP	serology +	3 U/kg/d i.v.	≥2	recovered		Ranze et al. [25]
26	M, 14 y, 26 kg	subdural hematoma, renal failure, dialysis		non-HIT	not done	mean prehemodialysis: 53 U/kg bolus i.v.	14	recovered		von Roth et al. [14]
27	M, 11 y 55 kg	iliac artery injury, compartment syndrome, renal failure, dialysis, postappendectomy		TP, ECC clots	serology +	prehemodialysis: 27 – 45 U/kg bolus i.v. + 2.7 U/kg/h	n/a	recovered		Lischetzki et al. [26]
28	F, 12 d	CHD		TP	serology –, clinical +	36 U/h	n/a	treatment withdrawal, died		Newall et al. [27]
29	M, 23 mo	acute metabolic decompensation		TP	serology +	for hemofiltration: 52 U/h	n/a	recovered		Newall et al. [27]
30	M, 2.5 mo	CHD (2 × CPBS), heart failure		TP, SVC thrombosis	not done	for SVC thrombectomy: 200 U/h i.v. infusion	n/a	persistent SVC thrombosis, died		Newall et al. [27]
31	M, 13 mo	CHD, renal agenesis, cardiac arrhythmia postsurgery		TP, right iliac artery thrombosis (catheter related)	serology +	n/a	n/a	n/a		Klenner et al. [29]
32	M, 15 mo	CHD, post-heart surgery		TP, effusions pleural/pericardial/ascites, peritonitis	serology +	n/a	5	recovered		Klenner et al. [29]
33	F, 15 y	brain biopsy, postoperative SSST		SSST extension to cavernous and straight sinuses	serology +	n/a	n/a	recovered		Klenner et al. [29]

ANA = Antinuclear antibody; APL = antiphospholipid syndrome; AST = aspartate aminotransferase; ATD = antithrombin deficiency; BW = body weight (kg); CHD = congenital heart disorder; CUP = compassionate use (named patient) program of NV Organon; d = days; ECC = extracorporeal circuit (for hemodialysis or hemofiltration); HLP IIa = hyperlipoproteinemia type IIa; ICT = intracardiac thrombus; IVC = inferior vena cava; mo = months; MOF = multiple organ failure; n/a = not available; PCD = protein C deficiency; PE = pulmonary embolism; PSD = protein S deficiency; RDS = respiratory distress syndrome; rt-PA = recombinant tissue plasminogen activator; SDH = subdural hematoma; SSST = sinus sagittalis superior thrombosis; SVC = superior vena cava; TE = thromboembolic event; TP = platelet count reduction/thrombocytopenia; VACTERL = syndrome of vertebral anomalies, anal atresia, cardiac anomalies, tracheo-esophageal fistula, renal anomalies and limb anomalies; y = years.

[a] Includes adverse events occurring within 1 month of danaparoid discontinuation.

Table 2. Summary statistics of demographic and presenting clinical features

Age and presenting clinical problems[a, b]	HIT	Non-HIT
Number of cases	33	1
Age		
Mean	8 years 7 months	
Median	10 years 5 months	14 years
Range	12 days to 17 years	
Thromboembolic event		
Preceding HIT	12	0
HIT complication	17	0
Any thrombotic/clotting event	21	0
Active bleeding	3	1
Clinical problem[c]		
Cardiac disease (congenital or acquired)	12	0
Intracardiac thrombus	3	0
Renal failure	6	1
Postoperative	13	0
Cancer	1	0
Hemostatic problem[d]		
PC/PS/AT deficiency	6	0
APL syndromes	8	0

PC = Protein C; PS = protein S; AT = antithrombin; APL = antiphospholipid syndrome.
[a] In 1 infant a pulmonary embolism was only suspected.
[b] A patient may have 1 or more of these clinical problems.
[c] A patient may have 1 or more of these hemostatic problems.
[d] Three patients had both PS or PC and APL syndromes.

ued with prophylactic use), anticoagulation for operations (all with cardiopulmonary bypass, CPB) in 5 cases, to protect extracorporeal circuits (5 for hemodialysis, 1 for hemofiltration) in 6 cases, peritoneal dialysis in 2 cases, cardiac catheterization in 1 case and as an intravenous line flush in 1 case. For 4 cases (No. 28, 31–33) the reason why danaparoid was given was not reported.

Diagnosis of HIT and Danaparoid Cross-Reactivity

For 29 of the 33 cases serological data for HIT diagnosis are available. Some were tested by more than one method. In 23 (including previous data for case 1 with past HIT) all tests were positive, and in 1 patient only 1 of 4 tests was positive. In 5 cases the serological tests were negative, but in 2 of these (No. 5 and 6) HIT was confirmed clinically after rechallenge resulting in thrombocytopenia. In the other 3 (No. 23, 24 and 28) HIT was strongly suspected clinically despite the negative laboratory tests. The method of HIT diagnosis is unknown for 3 patients (No. 11, 12 and 20) and 1 case was not tested (No. 30). Overall the diagnosis of HIT was confirmed serologically or clinically in 26/33 (78.8%) of the suspected HIT patients. Testing for pretreatment danaparoid cross-reactivity was reported for 12 of the 32 cases with confirmed or suspected acute HIT. Weak positive reactions in the ELISA test were recorded in 2 cases (No. 7 and 19); otherwise the remainder was negative in all tests but includes 1 case (No. 5) which was also negative for the HIT antibody.

Table 3. Thrombotic events at first presentation and during HIT

Type of thrombotic event[a]	Pre-HIT	HIT
DVT only	6	8
Pulmonary embolus only	0	2[b]
DVT and pulmonary embolus	4	1
Intracardiac thrombus	2	1
Peripheral arterial thrombus	2	3
Extracorporeal circuit clotting	0	4
Internal conduit clotting	0	1

[a] Some patients had more than 1 event.
[b] In 1 patient only suspected due to acute respiratory difficulty.

Thrombophilia and Thromboembolic Problems

Risk factors for thrombophilia, such as protein C, protein S or antithrombin deficiency, or antiphospholipid antibody syndromes or DIC (singly or in various combinations) were reported in 10/34 patients, but not all reports mentioned additional risk factors if any. Thromboembolic problems occurring prior to danaparoid therapy initiation are summarized in table 3. Thromboses mostly occurred within 2–7 days prior to danaparoid treatment initiation.

Factors at Presentation Increasing the Bleeding Risk

An increased bleeding risk prior to danaparoid treatment initiation was present in 10 patients who had undergone recent surgery: in 3 it was neurosurgery to excise a vascular malformation causing intracranial bleeding (No. 2) or to remove a subdural hematoma (No. 12 and 26, who also presented with renal failure). In 6 patients (No. 9, 10, 20, 24, 30 and 32) the surgery had been per-

Table 4. Comparison of pediatric and adult danaparoid dosing requirements

Clinical situation	Target anti-Xa activity	Pediatric age group[a]		Equivalent adult (70 kg) dose
		≤2 years	9–17 years	
Prophylaxis of TE	0.1–0.4 U/ml	8–144 U/kg/day	20–25 U/kg/day	21–32 U/kg/day
Treatment of TE	0.4–0.8 U/ml	no information	29–130 U/kg/day	69 U/kg/day
Cardiac catheterization	0.5–0.7 U/ml	48–120 U/kg/day	no information	36 U/kg i.v. bolus
Peritoneal dialysis	insufficient data	5–43 U/kg/day	no information	25 U/kg/day
Hemodialysis	0.5–0.8 U/ml	no information	27–86 U/kg bolus i.v.	43 U/kg/dialysis
Cardiac surgery	1.5–2.0 U/ml	350 U/kg/operation[b]	>150 U/kg[c] to ~311 U/kg/operation[d]	232 U/kg[e]

TE = Thromboembolic event.
[a] No patients with ages between 3 and 8 years inclusive.
[b] Assuming a 4-hour CPBS.
[c] Amount given intraoperatively not known.
[d] Assuming body weights of 33 and 45 kg, respectively, for the 2 cases.
[e] Assuming an average of 16,250 U danaparoid for CPBS.

formed using CPB. One patient had hepatic dysfunction after her second hepatic transplant (No. 21). Seven non-surgical patients had renal failure (No. 5, 6, 12, 19, 22, 27 and 29) and 1 patient (No. 8) with a rhabdomyosarcoma and chemotherapy-induced thrombocytopenia presented with epistaxis and petechiae.

Intensity and Duration of Danaparoid Use

Individual danaparoid regimens for each patient are shown in table 1 and are summarized in relation to target plasma anti-Xa activity levels in table 4. Most cases had regular plasma anti-Xa activity monitoring to maintain levels within the target ranges. For those cases whose published reports omitted proper dosing and/or body weight information, body weights were interpolated from the data provided for the rest of the cases (an S-shaped curve was fitted to the available data).

The duration of danaparoid use ranged from 1 day to 1.5 years (median 8 days). Danaparoid was stopped prematurely in 4 patients (cases 7, 13, 18 and 19, see below) because clinical cross-reactivity was suspected. In 4 patients (cases 4, 7, 23 and 34) danaparoid was used concomitantly with a thrombolytic (urokinase and/or rt-PA); 1 developed bleeding from venipuncture sites. In 8 patients (cases 2, 4, 9, 10, 13, 14, 15 and 16) danaparoid overlapped with VKA before withdrawal. No problem was reported with international normalized ratio measurements.

General Treatment Outcomes

General treatment outcomes and adverse events during danaparoid therapy are shown in table 1 and are summarized in table5. For case 31 no information is available [7, 29]. Adequate clinical outcomes of danaparoid use, based on the available data and as defined in the Methods section, were recorded for 22 patients (64.7% of all and 66.7% of those with outcome data available). Twenty-one of these (see table 5) had no or a minor adverse event without sequelae and patient 15, whose preexisting ischemia had not progressed during 30 days of danaparoid therapy, had some toes amputated after danaparoid treatment was completed by overlapping with a VKA [23]. No skin hypersensitivity or anaphylactic reactions were reported. Ten cases (described in the next section) suffered serious clinical events during danaparoid administration.

Adverse Events

Mortality

Five deaths (14.7% of all and 15.6% of those with known treatment outcome) were reported (No. 12, 21, 24, 28 and 30). Case 12, with CHD and renal failure, developed HIT after placement of two artificial heart valves. One valve clotted and a subdural hematoma developed. After failure to respond to thrombolytics she was started on danaparoid. Her valve function improved but after 8 days she died of a suspected pulmonary hemorrhage which if so can be attributed to the use of danaparoid [21]. Two other deaths can also be attributable to the danaparoid

Table 5. Danaparoid treatment outcomes

Diagnosis	Patient recovered			Patient death	
	no event/ minor event	major event sequelae	danaparoid prematurely stopped	TE or MB or unknown	other (MOF)
HIT confirmed	1, 2, 3, 4, 8, 9[b], 14, 16, 17, 22, 25, 27, 29, 32, 33, 34	15	7[c], 10[b], 13[c], 18[c], 19		21
HIT unconfirmed	5, 6, 11, 23		20[b]	12, 24[b], 28, 30[b]	
Non-HIT	26				
Total cases[a]	21	1	6	4	1

Apart from the row of total cases, numbers represent case No. TE = Thromboembolic event; MB = major bleed; MOF = multiple organ failure.

[a] For case 31 there is no information.

[b] Patients undergoing surgery with CPB.

[c] Cases 7, 13 and 18 were switched to lepirudin, for case 19 the new treatment is unknown.

treatment: case 24 developed fatal bleeding during a fourth thrombectomy with CPB to remove a thrombus on a mechanical heart valve (previously unpublished) and case 30, who had undergone 2 operations using CPB, died following rethrombosis of the superior vena cava after thrombectomy under danaparoid prophylaxis [27]. The deaths of cases 21 and 28 were probably not related to danaparoid treatment – case 21 (previously unpublished) died of sepsis and multiple organ failure 3 weeks after danaparoid treatment was discontinued and case 28 died after withdrawal of treatment for an unknown reason, but with no reported thrombotic or bleeding complications [27].

Thrombotic Events

Thrombosis (-related) events were reported in 5 cases (No. 13, 15, 19, 24 and 30). In case 13 [23] prior cardiac thrombi regressed during danaparoid therapy but a new DVT developed after 25 days of treatment without a platelet count reduction. The patient was switched to lepirudin, because clinical cross-reactivity was suspected but not serologically confirmed, and no further problem occurred. Case 15 [23] needing amputation is described above. Case 19 (previously unpublished) developed clotting in a hemodialysis circuit despite a high predialysis danaparoid dose. This was probably due to clinical cross-reactivity in view of the suspiciously positive PAT for pretreatment cross-reactivity and no dialysis was completed. Cases 24 and 30 [27] are described in the Mortality section.

Bleeding Events

Four major (No. 10, 12, 20 and 24) and 2 minor (No. 4 and 9) bleeding events were reported. Patient 10, who presented with coagulopathy before danaparoid treatment, bled severely following a Fontan procedure [28]. Altering the danaparoid infusion rate is reported to have had no influence on the bleeding rate which eventually stopped after 10 days despite continuation of the danaparoid infusion and the patient recovered. For details of case 12, see Mortality section above. Case 20 (previously unpublished) required large transfusions of blood, platelets and fresh frozen plasma before post-cardiopulmonary bypass surgery (post-CPBS) bleeding was brought under control. She had been transfused postsurgery with blood loss collected intraoperatively. For details of case 24, see Mortality section above. Case 4 bled from venipuncture sites during thrombolysis. The bleeding was controlled by stopping the thrombolytic, but the danaparoid infusion was continued [17]. Case 9 had a total post-CPBS blood loss of 700 ml [22].

Platelet Counts

Platelet counts recovered, as defined in the Methods section, in 18 of 19 patients (94.7%) with a low platelet count at danaparoid treatment initiation. Patient 18 developed a new platelet count reduction, despite receiving platelet transfusions, but a test for cross-reactivity was negative. At the time the infant had cytomegalovirus and *Klebsiella pneumoniae* infections. The patient was switched to lepirudin, but the thrombopenia persisted

[24]. Patient 21 developed a new thrombopenia during a stormy posthepatic transplant course which included sepsis, multiple organ failure and inadvertent catheter flushes with heparin. A new test for seroconversion was negative.

Other Adverse Events

Case 10 who underwent a second Fontan procedure on danaparoid had pretreatment hepatic thrombotic problems. Postoperatively she developed high AST and lactate levels, but these recovered during continued danaparoid therapy [28].

Danaparoid Cross-Reactivity and Suspected Seroconversion

Four patients (No. 7, 13, 18 and 19) developed or were suspected of clinical cross-reactivity. Case 7 presented with lower limb arterial and IVC thromboses complicating HIT. Although the platelet count increased, he was immediately switched to lepirudin when the weakly positive serological result became known on day 1 of danaparoid treatment. Despite adding urokinase an amputation was required 3 weeks later, following which further necrotic tissue was debrided [19]. Case 19 also showed weak serological cross-reactivity (see Thrombotic Events above). For the other 2 cases (case 13 [23]: see Thrombotic Events above and case 18 [24]: see Platelet Counts above) serological confirmation of cross-reactivity is lacking.

Discussion

Although uncommon in children HIT or other forms of (LMW) heparin intolerance can present a serious clinical problem. Part of the reason is the frequent association of HIT with diseases and/or disorders which further increase the thrombotic tendency, add a bleeding risk or otherwise compromise the clinical status of the patient [3]. Alternative antithrombotic treatment options are limited because effective drugs have not been specifically studied in subjects under the age of 18 years. Hence experience of danaparoid use in children, as for other antithrombotic alternatives, accumulates slowly as a result of case reports.

Assessment of the suitability of the various treatment alternatives for HIT is dependent on the quality and quantity of individual reports. This review is limited more by insufficient information (concerning important anamnestic details: demographic, temporal and clinical; details of danaparoid use including body weight, exact description of the dosage regimen and concomitant medication, and clinical outcome details) in the published reports than by the small number of reported cases treated with danaparoid.

Furthermore, clinical outcomes of danaparoid treatment have been assessed in several different ways. Most significantly, Klenner et al. [29] use the term 'survived' and add any adverse event which occurred, Zöhrer et al. [23] refer to 'clinical recovery', Ranze et al. [30] refer to 'positive outcome', while Newall et al. [27] describe the actual clinical events as do the reviews of Spinler and Dager [31] and Smythe [32] for adult treatment outcomes. These differences confuse collation and comparison of the reports of the available treatment options since both 'survived' and 'recovery' include certain clinical/adverse events subjectively and, as with mere descriptions of specific events, many do not take the individual clinical circumstances surrounding these events into account.

In addition, many reviews include both confirmed and suspected HIT cases, but Klenner and Greinacher [7] have recently argued against this and also included patients aged 18 years – whether this is justified or not remains to be proven. The 'routine' functional serological tests, particularly the PAT which is the most routinely available test, lack sensitivity especially when antibody titers are low in the early stages of HIT [33]. More sensitive tests, e.g. the EIA, may not be available and moreover not positive if the antibody is directed against a heparin-binding protein other than PF4. Thus tests in early HIT may be negative. This diagnostic uncertainty is highlighted by Schmugge et al. [6] and Donovan [34] and by Klenner and Greinacher [7] who cite, among others, the cases described by Neuhaus et al. [18] as unlikely to have HIT. Yet, despite negative results with both the HIPAA and EIA tests, these authors found rechallenge thrombocytopenia and dialysis circuit clotting in both patients with heparin but not with danaparoid. Diagnostic uncertainty and the high risk of thrombosis even after the causative drug has been discontinued [35] have led to the practice of initiating alternative antithrombotic therapy immediately if HIT is suspected even before any serological test result is available [36]. If the new treatment is successful but a pretreatment sample was serologically negative or not tested for HIT, then often no (further) diagnostic testing is performed.

In this review we identified 34 case reports of children aged 12 days to 17 years with diverse underlying clinical problems, who were treated with danaparoid. The diagnosis of HIT was serologically investigated in 29/33

(87.8%) of the reported cases and confirmed in 24/33 (72.7%). Although 9/33 patients (27.3%) did not meet the strict serological criteria for HIT according to Warkentin et al. [33], in all cases danaparoid was used by the treating physician because the clinical picture strongly suggested HIT. Therefore, for the purposes of this review the diagnosis of HIT mentioned in the case reports was accepted.

Survival analysis of danaparoid use identified 28 survivors (84.8%), 5 deaths (15.2%) and for 1 infant the outcome is unknown. These figures compare favorably with the outcomes reported by Klenner and Greinacher [7] of the fewer children treated with argatroban [i.e. 3 survivors (60%), 2 deaths, no outcomes unknown] or lepirudin [8 survivors (73%), 2 deaths, 1 outcome unknown], respectively.

An adequate clinical response to danaparoid, as defined in the Methods section, was found in 23 patients (67%). Nonfatal major adverse events occurred in 7 cases, 5 during and 2 after danaparoid use. One patient (No. 21) developed a new platelet count reduction after a catheter was flushed with unfractionated heparin. This patient's experience underlines the need to ensure elimination of all sources of the causative heparin in patients suffering from HIT. The 2 events in the danaparoid follow-up period were amputations (cases 7 and 15). This amputation frequency (5.8%) is within the range reported for adults and is similar to those reported by others for children suffering from HIT (~4% [29]). Of the 4 major bleeding events (cases 10, 12, 20 and 24) 3 occurred in the group of patients undergoing CPBS and 1 of these was fatal (case 24). Therefore, based on these few observations the use of danaparoid during CPBS cannot be recommended, which is in accordance with the observations in adults [36].

Of the 5 deaths 2 (5.9%) were unlikely to be due to the use of danaparoid (cases 21 and 28) but the other 3 (8.8%) can be linked to danaparoid use (cases 12, 24 and 30). Interestingly none of the deaths occurred in a confirmed HIT patient, but assuming that all patients had a correct diagnosis of HIT, then the overall mortality with danaparoid use is similar to that described by others for pediatric and adult HIT patients, i.e. 11.6% [7, 34].

The authors agree with Greinacher et al. [37] that ideally a pretreatment plasma sample should be tested for danaparoid cross-reactivity, but danaparoid can be started before the result is known. In the present review pretreatment danaparoid cross-reactivity was found in 2 of the 9 acute HIT patients tested. Treatment in both was started prior to the result being known, but both patients were switched to an alternative antithrombotic after 1 day, although only 1 developed renewed thrombotic problems. Two other patients were assumed to have seroconverted (cases 13 and 18) because of new clinical events, but serology was not performed in either case [23, 24]. Since other causes of new platelet count reduction/nonrecovery and new thromboembolic events during antithrombotic therapy can be present, e.g. sepsis, DIC, or other drugs, we recommend serological or skin testing for danaparoid cross-reactivity before treatment and repeated testing if seroconversion is suspected. If the result is positive, but the platelet count is recovering and there is no other evidence of clinical cross-reactivity, then danaparoid can be continued with daily platelet count monitoring. If clinical events are observed as a result of cross-reactivity, then it is important that these children are not exposed to danaparoid in the future.

Regular measurement of the plasma anti-Xa activity was reported in most cases, similar to the recommendations for the LMW heparins [38], i.e. daily for the first days, then twice weekly for the first weeks and later weekly to monthly intervals. Dosing intensity based on monitoring ensures that the target levels are not only reached but also maintained and not exceeded, especially if renal failure is present. Because of the few cases treated, their wide range of age and body weight and the variety of clinical indications for an antithrombotic no clear dosing recommendations can be given yet. However, the reviewed experience suggests that children below the age of 2 years may need higher doses of danaparoid per kilogram body weight to achieve the same target anti-Xa levels as children above 9 years or adults [39]. In general, the danaparoid regimens used remain similar to those recommended by Ranze and Greinacher [40], i.e. 2–10 U/kg b.d., s.c. for thromboprophylaxis and an intravenous bolus of 30 U/kg followed by an intravenous infusion of 29–96 U/kg/day (1.2–4.0 U/kg/h) for thrombosis treatment, but higher than the recommendations of Monagle et al. [41] to use 1.2–2.4 U/kg/h.

We recommend that when reporting the use of any drug in children the body weight, the complete dosing regimen and/or the total amount of drug administered for a specific procedure (e.g. perioperatively), the duration of use and a clear statement of the timing of clinical events in relation to the treatment should be provided. It would also be appropriate to report all adverse events with the above information directly to the drug manufacturer and to the national health institutions even if the case is independently published.

Conclusions

The HIT diagnosis remains difficult in some cases, but the high risk of a thrombotic problem makes switching to an alternative antithrombotic imperative when HIT is suspected.

This review of pediatric cases (aged 2 weeks to 17 years inclusive) finds that danaparoid can be used as an alternative antithrombotic agent in children with HIT or heparin intolerance. However, it cannot be recommended for surgery with CPB.

The dosing intensity in children should be guided by the plasma anti-Xa response, but the present limited information does not yet allow recommendation of optimal dosing regimens. Nevertheless, the data suggest that at least babies and infants require a higher dose per kilogram body weight than older children and adults to achieve the same plasma anti-Xa activity response and antithrombotic protection.

It is still not evident to what extent seroconversion with danaparoid is a problem since most cases in the adult literature and 3 of 4 suspected cases in this pediatric review were not confirmed serologically. However, from our personal experience and because of the potential clinical impact we recommend serological testing for cross-reactivity both before treatment and if clinical cross-reactivity is suspected.

Acknowledgements

The authors wish to thank Dr. H.J. Kreutzenbeck of Celltech Pharma GmbH, Essen, Germany for helpful advice and support. We also thank Dr. S. Doubine and Dr. P. Piquet (†) from Paris for the data concerning patient 24.

References

1 Magnani HN: Heparin-induced thrombocytopenia (HIT): an overview of 230 patients treated with organan (Org 10172). Thromb Haemost 1993;70:554–561.
2 Magnani HN: Orgaran (danaparoid) use in the syndrome of heparin-induced thrombocytopenia. Platelets 1997;8:74–81.
3 Risch L, Fischer JE, Herklotz R, Huber AR: Heparin-induced thrombocytopenia in paediatrics: clinical characteristics, therapy and outcome. Intensive Care Med 2004;30:1615–1624.
4 Warkentin TE: Heparin-induced thrombocytopenia: pathogenesis and management. Br J Haematol 2003;121:535–555.
5 Warkentin TE, Roberts RS, Hirsh J, Kelton JG: An improved definition of immune heparin-induced thrombocytopenia in postoperative orthopedic patients. Arch Intern Med 2003;163:2815–2824.
6 Schmugge M, Risch L, Huber AR, Benn A, Fischer JE: Heparin-induced thrombocytopenia-associated thrombosis in pediatric intensive care patients. Pediatrics 2002;109:E10.
7 Klenner AF, Greinacher A: Heparin-induced thrombocytopenia in children; in Warkentin TE, Greinacher A (eds): Heparin-Induced Thrombocytopenia, ed 3. New York, Marcel Dekker, 2004, pp 553–571.
8 Chong BH, Castaldi PA: Heparin-induced thrombocytopenia: further studies of the effects of heparin-dependent antibodies on platelets. Br J Haematol 1986;64:347–354.
9 Greinacher A, Michels I, Mueller-Eckhardt C: Heparin-associated thrombocytopenia: successful therapy of patients after prospective selection of a compatible heparinoid with the heparin-induced platelet activation test (in German). Beitr Infusionsther 1992;30:408–412.
10 Amiral J, Bridey F, Wolf M, Boyer-Neumann C, Fressinaud E, Vissac AM, Peynaud-Debayle E, Dreyfus M, Meyer D: Antibodies to macromolecular platelet factor 4-heparin complexes in heparin-induced thrombocytopenia: a study of 44 cases. Thromb Haemost 1995;73:21–28.
11 Sheridan D, Carter C, Kelton JG: A diagnostic test for heparin-induced thrombocytopenia. Blood 1986;67:27–30.
12 Girisch M, Buheitel G, Ries M, Klinge J: Safe and effective use of danaparoid during cardiac catheterization in a 14 month old boy with tetralogy of Fallot and heparin-induced thrombocytopenia (abstract 68). Ann Hematol 2001; 80(suppl):A20.
13 Teien AN, Lie M: Evaluation of an amidolytic heparin assay method: increased sensitivity by adding purified antithrombin III. Thromb Res 1977;10:399–410.
14 von Roth B, Herkenrath P, Krebber J, Anschütz K: Use of a new heparinoid as the sole anticoagulant in haemodialysis of paediatric patients (in German). Nieren Hochdruckkrankheiten 1985;14:164.
15 Barth KSA: Incidence of the Heparin-Induced Thrombocytopenia at the Justus Liebig University Hospital (in German); MD thesis Justus Liebig University, Giessen, 1998.
16 Bocquet R, Blanot S, Dautzenberg MD, Pierre-Kahn A, Carli P: Antiphospholipid antibody syndrome in pediatric neurosurgery: a haemostasis problem (in French). Ann Fr Anesth Reanim 1999;18:991–995.
17 Klement D, Rammos S, von Kries R, Kirschke W, Kniemeyer HW, Greinacher A: Heparin as a cause of thrombus progression. Heparin-associated thrombocytopenia is an important differential diagnosis in paediatric patients even with normal platelet counts. Eur J Pediatr 1996;155:11–14.
18 Neuhaus TJ, Goetschel P, Schmugge M, Leumann E: Heparin-induced thrombocytopenia type II on haemodialysis: switch to danaparoid. Pediatr Nephrol 2000;14:713–716.
19 Schiffmann H, Unterhalt M, Harms K, Figulla HR, Völpel H, Greinacher A: Successful treatment of heparin-induced thrombocytopenia (HIT) type II in childhood with recombinant hirudin (in German). Monatsschr Kinderheilkd 1997;145:606–612.
20 Sauer M, Gruhn B, Fuchs D, Altermann W, Zintl F: Heparin-induced thrombocytopenia type II during high-dose chemotherapy with stem-cell-rescue (in German). Klin Pädiatr 1998;210:102–105.
21 Weigel B, Laskey A, Krishnamurti L, Perentesis J, Neglia J, Foker J, Key N, Edson R, Steiner M: Danaparoid (orgaran) anticoagulation of pediatric patients with heparin-induced thrombocytopenia. J Pediatr Hematol Oncol 1999;321:327.
22 Wilhelm MJ, Schmid C, Kececioglu D, Mollhoff T, Ostermann H, Scheld HH: Cardiopulmonary bypass in patients with heparin-induced thrombocytopenia using Org 10172. Ann Thorac Surg 1996;61:920–924.
23 Zöhrer B, Zenz W, Rettenbacher A, Covi P, Kurnik K, Kroll H, Grubbauer HM, Muntean W: Danaparoid sodium (Orgaran) in four children with heparin-induced thrombocytopenia type II. Acta Paediatr 2001;90:765–771.

24 Nguyen TN, Gal P, Ransom JL, Carlos R: Lepirudin use in a neonate with heparin-induced thrombocytopenia. Ann Pharmacother 2003; 37:229–233.
25 Ranze O, Rakow A, Ranze P, Eichler P, Greinacher A, Fusch C: Low-dose danaparoid sodium catheter flushes in an intensive care infant suffering from heparin-induced thrombocytopenia. Pediatr Crit Care Med 2001;2: 175–177.
26 Lischetzki G, Dittrich K, Topf H-G, Klinge J: Pediatric heparin-induced thrombocytopenia type II on haemodialysis (abstract P38). Haemostaseologie 2004;24:A48.
27 Newall F, Barnes C, Ignjatovic V, Monagle P: Heparin-induced thrombocytopenia in children. J Paediatr Child Health 2003;39:289–292.
28 Saxon BR, Black MD, Edgell D, Noel D, Leaker MT: Pediatric heparin-induced thrombocytopenia: management with danaparoid (Orgaran). Ann Thorac Surg 1999;68:1076–1078.
29 Klenner AF, Lubenow N, Raschke R, Greinacher A: Heparin-induced thrombocytopenia in children: 12 new cases and a review of the literature. Thromb Haemost 2004;91:719–724.
30 Ranze O, Ranze P, Magnani HN, Greinacher A: Heparin-induced thrombocytopenia in paediatric patients: a review of the literature and a new case treated with danaparoid sodium. Eur J Paediatr 1999;158(suppl 3):S130–S133.
31 Spinler SA, Dager W: Overview of heparin-induced thrombocytopenia. Am J Health Syst Pharm 2003;60:S5–S11.
32 Smythe M: A comparison of argatroban and lepirudin outcomes (abstract). Thromb Haemost 2003;1(suppl 1):P2041.
33 Warkentin TE: Platelet count monitoring and laboratory testing for heparin-induced thrombocytopenia. Arch Pathol Lab Med 2002;126; 1415–1423.
34 Donovan PC: Heparin-induced thrombocytopenia: strategies for identification and treatment. Clin Rev 2001;11:93–105.
35 Warkentin TE: Clinical picture of HIT; in Warkentin TE, Greinacher A (eds): Heparin-Induced Thrombocytopenia, ed 3. New York, Marcel Dekker, 2004, pp 53–106.
36 Warkentin TE, Greinacher A: Heparin-induced thrombocytopenia and cardiac surgery. Ann Thorac Surg 2003;76:2121–2131.
37 Greinacher A, Lubenow N, Hinz P, Ekkernkamp A: Heparin-induced thrombocytopenia (in German). Dtsch Ärztebl 2003;100:2220–2229.
38 Albisetti M, Andrew M: Low molecular weight heparin in children. Eur J Pediatr 2002;161: 71–77.
39 Greinacher A, Warkentin TW: Treatment of heparin-induced thrombocytopenia; in Warkentin TE, Greinacher A (eds): Heparin-Induced Thrombocytopenia, ed 3. New York, Marcel Dekker, 2004, pp 335–370.
40 Ranze O, Greinacher A: Current treatment concepts in heparin-induced thrombocytopenia (in German). Dtsch Med Wochenschr 1999;124:865–873.
41 Monagle P, Michelson AD, Bovill E, Andrew M: Antithrombotic therapy in children. Chest 2001;119(1 suppl):344S–370S.

Acta Hæmatologica

Author Index Vol. 115, No. 3–4, 2006

Subject Index Vol. 115, No. 3–4, 2006

KARGER
Fax +41 61 306 12 34
E-Mail karger@karger.ch
www.karger.com

Accessible online at:
www.karger.com/aha

Author Index Vol. 115, 2006

Acta Hæmatologica

KARGER

Fax +41 61 306 12 34
E-Mail karger@karger.ch
www.karger.com

Accessible online at:
www.karger.com/aha

Subject Index Vol. 115, 2006

Acta Haematologica

KARGER

Fax +41 61 306 12 34
E-Mail karger@karger.ch
www.karger.com

Accessible online, at
www.karger.com/aha

Vol. 115, 2006

Acta Hæmatologica

Founded 1948 by E. Meulengracht, K. Rohr, and G. Rosenow
Continued by H. Lüdin (1960–1977), U. Bucher (1977–1983), R.S. Hillman (1978–1987), H.R. Marti (1983–1988), E.A. Beck (1984–1988), B. Ramot (1989–1995)

KARGER

Basel · Freiburg · Paris · London · New York ·
Bangalore · Bangkok · Singapore · Tokyo · Sydney

S. Karger
Medical and Scientific Publishers
Basel • Freiburg • Paris • London
New York • Bangalore • Bangkok
Singapore • Tokyo • Sydney

Printed in Switzerland on acid-free paper by
Reinhardt Druck, Basel

KARGER

Fax +41 61 306 12 34
E-Mail karger@karger.ch
www.karger.com

Acta Hæmatologica

Contents Vol. 115, 2006

No. 1–2

Review

Original Papers

Case Reports

Brief Communications

KARGER

Fax +41 61 306 12 34
E-Mail karger@karger.ch
www.karger.com

Access to full text and tables of contents, including tentative ones for forthcoming issues: www.karger.com/aha_issues

No. 3–4

Issues of Haemostasis and Thrombosis in Children

Guest Editors: Gili Kenet (Tel Hashomer); Ulrike Nowak-Göttl (Münster)